Overseas Doctors
in the
National Health Service

David J Smith

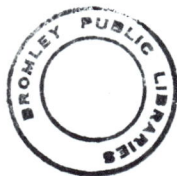

First published 1980

ISBN 0 435 83800 8

Printed and bound by George Berridge & Co. Ltd.
London & Thetford.

Acknowledgements

The study of overseas doctors in the National Health Service on which this report is based was financed by the Department of Health and Social Security. The study was designed after consultation with the Department, the Overseas Doctors' Association and the British Medical Association, and these three bodies were later invited to comment on the draft report. I am also grateful to the Council for Postgraduate Medical Education for help and advice.

Five of the case studies of hospitals were carried out by Naomi Connelly, whose general contribution to Chapter IX was at least as great as mine.

Piloting, fieldwork and pre-computer analysis was carried out by British Market Research Bureau (BMRB) Ltd. I am especially grateful to Graham Read and Ned Scott at BMRB who looked after this difficult project.

The test of colloquial English incorporated in the survey was developed after consultation with Joy Parkinson of Southwark College. Much of the material for test items was taken from 'A Manual of English for the Overseas Doctor' by Joy Parkinson, published by Churchill Livingstone in 1976. I am very grateful to Joy Parkinson for her help and for permission to use this material in the test.

The sample selection depended on the co-operation of 49 Area Health Authorities and 14 Regional Health Authorities in the National Health Service, and I would like to thank these Authorities for their help.

My special thanks go to Dr M E Abrams of the Department of Health and Social Security, whose constructive criticism has been extremely helpful to me, especially since he has never made any attempt to impose his own or the Department's views.

Contents

List of Tables in the Text

xi

I   Introduction

Since the 1950s, doctors from overseas have formed a substantial proportion of medical manpower in the National Health Service: they now
account for about one-third of hospital doctors and one-fifth of general
practitioners.[1] Most of these doctors had their basic training and obtained their basic qualification in the country of origin, but came to the UK
to complete their training and with the intention of returning to the country of origin after a few years. This pattern of migration was made possible because basic qualifications granted by a large number of foreign
medical colleges (including many in the Indian sub-continent) were
recognised by the British authority (the General Medical Council) for the
purpose of registration to practice in the UK. Further, while immigration
has been subject to increasingly strict controls from 1962 onwards, these
immigration controls have never been extended to qualified doctors. In
these ways, successive governments, by their immigration policies, and
the medical profession, by its registration policies, have made it possible
for overseas doctors to come to the UK.

In the absence of serious restraints, a substantial migration of doctors
from overseas was brought about by a demand for doctors in the
National Health Service (NHS) which could not be met by the British
medical schools. This excess demand arose because of the shortcomings
of medical manpower forecasting. The Willink report of 1957[2] greatly
underestimated future medical manpower requirements, and these low
estimates determined the output from British medical schools over the
following fifteen years. The resulting shortfall was made good by an influx of doctors from overseas. Thus, the influx was not planned, but, on
the contrary arose from a failure of planning.

The flow of overseas doctors had important implications for career
structures in the NHS, and consequently for training arrangements.
Because most overseas doctors came to this country for a limited period
early in their careers, they are heavily concentrated in the lower hospital
grades. In effect, the NHS can rely on a continually renewed pool of

---

1 On the basis of country of birth, according to DHSS statistics.
2 Report of the Committee to Consider the Future Numbers of Medical Practitioners and
Appropriate Intake of Medical Students, HMSO, London, (1957).

overseas doctors to fill a large proportion of junior hospital jobs. As long as these doctors leave before becoming consultants, an unusual career structure can be maintained in which junior doctors in training greatly outnumber consultants, yet British junior doctors still have reasonable prospects of reaching consultant status by the age of 35 or so.

The migration developed naturally out of Britain's historical links with ex-colonial territories. The hospital services in India, for example, were established by a British administration on the British pattern, and were later extended from this base by the independent government. Interchange of doctors between Britain and India has taken place for at least a hundred years. As the health services in India have expanded since independence, Indian doctors have naturally thought first of Britain as a country in which to gain experience and training, because of the historical ties between the two countries, because medical education in India is carried out in English and because the hospital system and the medical approach in India are modelled on the British pattern.

In the early 1970s, recognition that the shortage of British-trained doctors was persisting and ought to be corrected was accompanied by increasing doubts about the competence of Indian and other overseas doctors. In the sending countries, large numbers of new hospitals and medical colleges were being created about which the British authorities knew little. Whether standards of training at these many institutions were comparable with British ones it was difficult or impossible to establish. It was believed that some or many overseas doctors were handicapped by inadequate or idiosyncratic English. Any extra burden imposed by training an overseas compared with a British doctor became serious when one half of junior hospital doctors were from overseas. Relations between overseas doctors and their patients might sometimes be difficult, either because of a cultural or linguistic gap, or because of a degree of reserve or prejudice on the part of the patients.

These doubts on the part of the British medical profession were given official expression by the Committee of Inquiry into the Regulation of the Medical Profession (the Merrison Committee)[3] which, reporting in 1975, concluded that 'there are substantial numbers of overseas doctors whose skill and the care they offer fall below that generally acceptable in this country and it is at least possible that there are some who should not have been registered'. In accordance with the recommendations of the Committee, most doctors applying for temporary registration were now required to pass the TRAB examination[4] covering knowledge of English and of medicine. Doctors from countries with which the UK had reciprocal arrangements and whose qualifications were recognised for the purpose were still eligible for full registration and would not have to

---

[3] Report of the Committee of Inquiry into the Regulation of the Medical Profession, HMSO, London, (1975).
[4] The initials TRAB stand for Temporary Registration Assessment Board, the body that was set up to administer the examination.

take a further examination. At one time such reciprocal arrangements existed with most Commonwealth and ex-Commonwealth countries, but these had already ceased in the case of a number of countries (such as various Provinces of Canada, Pakistan and Sri Lanka) by the time that the Merrison Committee reported. Full registration could still be (and was) granted but from 1975 onwards, a substantial proportion of overseas doctors who wished to come to the UK, being eligible only for temporary registration, were required to take the TRAB examination.

There were also doubts on the part of overseas doctors as to whether they benefited from working and training in the UK as much as they had expected, or as much as they ought to do. Following the publication of the Merrison report, the Overseas Doctors Association was formed, and soon began to make criticisms of the treatment of overseas doctors, and to put forward recommendations. It was suggested that overseas doctors faced a number of difficulties which the NHS had done little to remedy. Unable to find a suitable job in the specialty of their choice, they were often forced to switch to a less popular one. Consequently, there was a marked concentration of overseas doctors in geriatrics and psychiatry, two specialties in which imperfect understanding of English and distance from British culture would be a particularly important handicap. Even when they had switched specialty, it was said that overseas doctors tended to find themselves in jobs in which hours were long and training opportunities poor. Because of these disadvantages, many did not complete their training, or pass their examinations, within the schedule they had set themselves; as difficulty hardened into failure, they would be less and less likely to return to their countries of origin because they had not obtained the qualifications for which they had come to Britain.

To the extent that these criticisms were justified, it would also follow that the health services of the sending countries were not benefiting from using the NHS as a training ground as much as they might have expected. A proportion of their doctors would return untrained and without suitable qualifications, or with training in second-choice specialties (such as geriatrics or psychiatry) having comparatively little relevance to developing countries, and a proportion would not return at all. Even those trained in a suitable specialty and who did return might find that the style of medicine that they had acquired was more appropriate to a developed than to a developing country.

In some respects, then, the unplanned intake of overseas doctors into the NHS looks like an arrangement that is mutually beneficial to the NHS, to the overseas doctors themselves, and to the medical services in the countries from which they come. In other respects, it can be argued that it works to the mutual disadvantage of all three parties. There can be little useful discussion of these questions, and of the policy issues that spring from them, without a more solid basis of fact. The Merrison report, although it recommended that changes should immediately be made in registration procedures, also recognised that the formation of policy was hampered by a lack of facts, and it recommended that a study of the experience of overseas doctors within the NHS should be carried out. The Overseas Doctors Association supported this recommendation, and the Department of Health and Social Security asked PEP (Political and Economic Planning, now the Policy Studies Institute) to undertake the present study.

Objectives

In carrying out a study of overseas doctors, it is difficult to take full account of the dimension of time. Ideally, there would be a historical treatment of the development of the migration. This can no longer be adequately done, because too little information was collected in the past. The whole group of overseas doctors now in Britain comprises people at every different stage of their careers. A rigorous comparative study of the experience of overseas and indigenous doctors would identify groups of doctors at the point where they obtained their basic qualifications and follow them through. However, such a study would take many years to complete, whereas the policy issues are pressing and urgent. Furthermore, a 'cohort' study of this kind, if started in 1977, would provide information not about the factors that have governed the career and training opportunities of the great majority of overseas doctors who are now working in the NHS, but about the experience of overseas doctors in the future.

Instead, this study was designed to describe and analyse the present experience of a cross section of all overseas doctors now in the UK, to make appropriate comparisons with the experience of indigenous doctors, and to interpret doctors' present experience, as far as possible, in the light of their career histories up to the present. This was achieved by interviewing a representative sample of overseas and indigenous doctors and questioning them about both their present and past experience.

From the findings of this survey we can make useful comparisons of career progress between overseas and indigenous doctors, taking into account differences in qualifications and knowledge of medical and colloquial English. (It is not, of course, possible to take into account medical competence, which cannot be assessed from a questionnaire survey). In addition, we can analyse the factors that influence the decision to remain in this country, to return to the country of origin, or to go on to another country. Also, detailed information can be provided on a wide range of topics, such as doctors' views of the fairness of selection procedures used by hospitals and general practices, and the nature and quality of relationships between overseas and indigenous doctors.

Method

A representative sample of 1,981 doctors in the NHS was selected and these doctors were interviewed between September 1977 and February 1978.

The survey was confined to England. Both general practitioners and hospital doctors were included. Certain minor groups were excluded (doctors with honorary contracts, those in the Blood Transfusion Service and Mass Radiography Units, general practitioners' assistants and trainees).

At the first stage of sampling, 50 Health Districts were selected, after stratification, from the 206 in England, with equal probabilities. Lists of all general practitioners and of all hospital doctors actually working in these districts were then established from NHS records, doctors born in Britain or Ireland being shown separately from those born elsewhere. The final sample was then randomly selected from these lists.

The numbers of overseas-born doctors selected were artificially boosted by a factor of about 4½ to 1, but population proportions were restored by weighting at the analysis stage. Thus, the final sample is representative of all doctors in the NHS (except for the minor excluded categories), but still contains a large enough number of overseas doctors for separate analysis.

Interviewing was carried out at hospitals and surgeries. The response rate achieved was 75 per cent for hospital doctors and 62 per cent for general practitioners. The sample profile can be compared with DHSS statistics (see Appendix B) and these comparisons show that the sample is closely representative of the population sampled.

Interviewing was carried out by the fieldforce of British Market Research Bureau Ltd. The hour-long questionnaire was developed through two stages of piloting. It was a structured questionnaire, that is, the exact wording of every question, and the exact sequence of questions, were specified; but a considerable number of open-ended questions were included.

In addition to the survey, informal investigations were carried out at nine hospitals, chosen to exemplify some of the main types, including teaching hospitals, general hospitals, psychiatric hospitals and geriatric hospitals. The nine hospitals were also geographically spread over the main regions of England. At each hospital informal interviews were carried out with a range of doctors in different grades and specialties including some from Britain and some from overseas. In addition, information was obtained about the structure and organization of the hospital from administrative staff.

Technical details and a copy of the survey questionnaire are contained in Appendix B and Appendix C.

A note on definitions and sources

This report is about working hospital doctors, and general practitioners who are unrestricted principals, in the NHS in England. There is a considerable number of doctors, for example, in teaching and research, who have honorary contracts allowing them to treat patients in a hospital, but who do not principally function as hospital doctors; they are not included in the subject matter of this report. There is also an appreciable number of general practitioners at an early stage of their careers who are acting as trainees or assistants (and not as unrestricted principals); this group, which accounts for two per cent of all general practitioners, is not covered in this report. The term 'all doctors' will be used to mean that great majority of all NHS doctors who were covered by our inquiry.

Comparisons between DHSS statistics and the PSI survey, which are shown in the Appendix B, show no significant differences. To avoid confusion, survey statistics will be used where possible; these may differ from the DHSS statistics by one or two percentage points.

Presentation and layout

The final chapter of this report (Chapter X) contains a summary of the main findings and a discussion of the policy implications. The reader who does not wish to read the report straight through should probably turn to the final chapter, and follow up more detailed points in the rest of the report afterwards.

There are two separate series of tables. The main series, numbered within chapters, are presented in the text close to the points where they are discussed. The additional tables, numbered from A1 to A50, are collected together in a separate section at the end of the report (Appendix A Additional Tables, p.206). All of these additional tables are used at some point in the text and a reference is given to the appropriate table, but the report can be read without consulting them.

In all the tables, an asterisk (*) is used to mean a quantity greater than 0 but less than 0.5 per cent. The sign for nil, or an empty cell, is a dash (—). In some of the Appendix and text tables, n.a. is used to indicate that the numbers involved were too low to be analysed. In most tables, the bases for percentages, that is, the totals on which percentages are calculated, are shown. It is a consequence of the sample design that all analysis must be carried out on weighted figures. Weighted and unweighted bases are normally shown. The weighted base is the base actually used for percentages, and reflects true population proportions. The unweighted base is the actual number of people included in a column, and gives the best indication of the accuracy of the results.

United Kingdom (or UK) has been used throughout the text and in the tables to denote the geographical area. The term 'British-qualified' includes, however, doctors who obtained their qualifications either in the United Kingdom or in Eire.

Percentages are rounded to the nearest whole number, so that columns may add slightly over or under the expected figure. Not all columns are expected to add to 100; in particular, there were many questions to which informants could give more than one answer, so that the percentages in these tables will add to more than 100.

Where the wording of a question was particularly important, the exact words used are shown with the table. In other cases, a reference to the question number (as 'Q33a') will normally be given. These references can be followed up by consulting the questionnaire reproduced in Appendix C.

Although this report shows 129 tables, these are a small selection of all the tabulations available. Also, further tabulations could be done. The reader who wishes to consult other tables, or who is interested in having further tabulations done, should get in touch with the author at the Policy Studies Institute.

II A General Description of British and Overseas Doctors

Country of origin

Nearly one-third of the survey population of doctors (31 per cent) were born outside the United Kingdom. Generally speaking, overseas doctors come to the UK for a period of training and experience in the hospital service, and many then return to the country of origin; among the

Table II.1   Country of birth of general practitioners and hospital doctors

Column Percentages

	All doctors	General practitioners	Hospital doctors
United Kingdom or Eire	69	80	62
of which			
United Kingdom	*67*	*76*	*60*
Eire	*2*	*4*	*2*
Other European countries	3	3	4
White anglophone countries[1]	3	2	3
Indian sub-continent	17	12	20
of which			
India	*12*	*10*	*14*
Pakistan	*2*	*1*	*2*
Bangladesh	*1*	*1*	*1*
Sri Lanka	*2*	*1*	*3*
Arab countries/Iran	3	1	5
African countries[2]	1	1	1
Far Eastern countries[3]	2	1	2
Other countries	2	1	2
Base: All informants			
Unweighted	*1,981*	*730*	*1,251*
Weighted	*4,490*	*1,923*	*2,567*

[1] Australia, New Zealand, South Africa, Rhodesia, USA and Canada
[2] Kenya, Uganda, Zambia, Tanzania, Malawi.
[3] Japan, Malaysia, Hong Kong, Taiwan

relatively small proportion who remain here indefinitely, some eventually become general practitioners (GPs). It is natural to find, therefore, that a higher proportion of hospital doctors (38 per cent) than of GPs (20 per cent) are overseas-born.

Overseas doctors come from a wide range of countries, among which the Indian sub-continent forms the most important group, accounting for 17 per cent of all doctors and for 20 per cent of hospital doctors (classified by country of birth). White anglophone countries (Australia, USA, Canada, South Africa and Rhodesia) account for 3 per cent of all doctors and Arab Countries for a further 3 per cent.

Table II.2 Relation between country of birth and country of first qualification: all doctors

		Percentages
	Born in UK/Eire	Born outside UK/Eire
First qualified in UK/Eire	69	6
First qualified outside UK/Eire	1	24

For most purposes it will be more relevant to define country of origin in terms of the country in which the doctor obtained his first basic medical qualification (the MB (Bachelor of Medicine) or equivalent). Country of birth and country of first qualification are strongly related, but do not quite amount to the same thing. The great majority of doctors (93 per cent) were born and first qualified in the same country, but there is a significant minority who were born overseas but came to the UK to go to medical school and first qualified here (6 per cent). These doctors will generally be classified as British rather than overseas doctors in this report.

Table II.3 Country of first qualification of general practitioners and hospital doctors

				Column percentages		
	All doctors		GPs		Hospital doctors	
United Kingdom or Eire	75		86		68	
White anglophone country	2		1		3	
Indian sub-continent	17	25	11	14	21	32
Arab countries	3		*		4	
Elsewhere (or not stated)	3		2		4	
Base: All informants						
Unweighted	*1,981*		*730*		*1,251*	
Weighted	*4,490*		*1,923*		*2,567*	

9

The classification by country of first qualification that will generally be used is shown in Table II.3. On this definition, 32 per cent of hospital doctors and 14 per cent of GPs are overseas-qualified.

The structure of our whole population can briefly be summarised as follows.

Per cent of all doctors:	
General practitioners	43
Hospital doctors	57
Per cent of general practitioners:	
Overseas-qualified	14
Overseas-born	20
Per cent of hospital doctors:	
Overseas-qualified	32
Overseas-born	38

Race or colour
On the basis of an interviewers' assessment of race or colour, 24 per cent of all doctors are non-white. The great majority of overseas doctors are coloured or black (86 per cent of overseas-qualified doctors, 77 per cent of overseas-born doctors). More detailed analyses are shown in Appendix Tables A1 and A2.

Age, sex and marital status
We shall see when doctors' career paths are analysed that general practice and the hospital service are two highly distinct medical careers which start from a common point. Most doctors spend at least two years in the hospital service after passing the Bachelor of Medicine examinations (MB)[1]. Thus, any cohort of doctors remains in the hospital service up to two years from the date of qualification, but from that time onwards, initially substantial and subsequently decreasing numbers peel off every year into general practice. After about ten years, the division into GPs and long-term hospital doctors is more or less complete. Thus, the general practice career starts after a period of training, or sometimes an attempted career, in the hospital service. It follows that GPs tend to be older than hospital doctors. In fact, only four per cent of the GPs in our sample (all of them unrestricted principals) were aged up to 29, compared with as many as 29 per cent of the hospital doctors.

Overseas doctors usually migrate to this country after practising for some years in their country of origin, so that comparatively few of them are aged under 30; and by the age of 44 they tend either to return to the

---

1 Those seeking full registration must spend at least one year, and it is usual for future general practitioners to spend at least one further year, in the hospital service.

country of origin or to move out of the hospital service to become GPs in the UK. Consequently, there is a strong tendency for overseas-qualified hospital doctors to fall within the 30 to 44 age group (A.3): 69 per cent are aged 30 to 44, compared with 33 per cent of British-qualified hospital doctors.

Overseas-qualified GPs are also concentrated in a middle age range (A.3), but at the upper end, i.e. from 35 to 54; 81 per cent are within this age range, compared with only 57 per cent of British qualified GPs. There are few young overseas-qualified GPs, because overseas doctors become GPs in this country only after completing some years in the hospital service, first in the country of origin and then here. There are comparatively few older overseas-qualified GPs because migration on a large scale began comparatively recently, and most migrants were aged around thirty when they came to the UK.

Women account for 16 per cent of all doctors, and the balance of the sexes is exactly the same among overseas-qualified and British-qualified doctors. Thirty-seven per cent of all women doctors are unmarried (A.4), compared with 11 per cent of men. Because of their relative youth, hospital doctors are more likely to be unmarried than GPs. Allowing for this, the proportions of overseas-qualified and British-qualified doctors who are unmarried are fairly similar, and this applies equally to both sexes.

Type of registration
At the time of the study (1977-78) the General Medical Council granted three kinds of registration for medical practice in the UK: provisional, temporary and full. Provisional registration is the kind normally held by British-qualified doctors during their first year of practice after obtaining the primary qualification (the MB or equivalent). After this first year as a house officer in the hospital service doctors are normally eligible for full registration. Overseas-qualified doctors whose primary qualification is recognised for the purpose of full registration may also qualify for provisional registration, although it is more usual for them to complete the equivalent of a first year as house officer in the country of origin, so that on coming to Britain they will be eligible for full registration.

Full registration is the only kind that places no limitations on the doctor's freedom to practice in any capacity. The requirements are a recognised primary medical qualification and practical experience as defined by the General Medical Council (GMC), that is, broadly of the kind that a British doctor obtains during his first 'pre-registration' year as a house officer. At the time of the study, primary qualifications recognised for the purpose of full registration, apart from the British ones, were those granted by certain medical colleges and universities in Australia, Canada, New Zealand, Hong Kong, Malaysia, Malta, Singapore, the West Indies, Burma and South Africa. Pakistani qualifications were recognised for full registration until 1972, when

Pakistan left the Commonwealth. Indian qualifications were recognised until May 1975, and those granted up to then were still recognised. The position was similar for Sri Lanka (up to the end of 1971) and Uganda (up to November 1976).

At the time of this study, temporary registration was the only kind that might be available to overseas-qualified doctors whose primary qualifications were not recognised for full registration — for example, to Indians who qualified after May 1975. This kind of registration (now superseded) imposed some limitations on the doctor's freedom to prac-tise. The temporarily registered doctor was entitled to work in a specified post for a specified period; the registration attached to that particular post, and the doctor had to be accepted for that post before applying for temporary registration. If he remained in the post for more than 12 months, he had to apply again at the end of that period for temporary registration. Since temporary registration was not available for posts in general practice, temporarily registered doctors were confined. to the hospital service.

Table II.4   Temporary registration among overseas-qualified
hospital doctors, by grade of post

Percentages

	Total	Grade of post:		
		HO/SHO[1]/ Registrar	SR/MA[2]	Consultant
Now temporarily registered	37	45	16	10
Temporarily registered in first post in the UK	45	50	24	33
Base: Overseas-qualified hospital doctors				
Unweighted	*712*	*544*	*59*	*85*
Weighted	*834*	*617*	*87*	*101*

1 House officer, senior house officer,
2 Senior registrar, medical assistant

Temporary registration was granted at the discretion of the GMC, which did not publish a full list of primary qualifications recognised for this purpose. However, it was stated in the Medical Register that Indian, Pakistani and Sri Lankan qualifications which were formerly recognised for the purpose of full registration were later recognised for temporary registration; in practice, qualifications from about 90 other countries were also recognised for temporary registration. From 1975, it was a re-quirement that applicants for temporary registration should have passed the TRAB examination (covering medical knowledge and knowledge of the English language), although some applicants were exempted.

Temporary registration was supposed to be for a person who intended to be in the United Kingdom temporarily. In the context of the employment for which he was temporarily registered, a temporarily registered doctor was on the same footing as a fully registered doctor. The registration was temporary in the sense that it had to be renewed and might, if the GMC so decided, be withdrawn. However, a substantial number of doctors worked as temporarily registered doctors for many years, and became senior within the hospital service. Table II.4 shows that while junior doctors were much more likely to be temporarily registered than senior ones, nevertheless 15 per cent of overseas-qualified senior registrars and medical assistants and 10 per cent of overseas-qualified consultants were temporarily registered. One-third of overseas-qualified consultants were temporarily registered in their first medical post in the UK, but 23 per cent subsequently obtained full registration, leaving only 10 per cent who were still temporarily registered at the time of the survey.

Among overseas-qualified hospital doctors generally, we find that 62 per cent had full registration at the time of the survey, 37 per cent had temporary registration and one per cent provisional registration. By comparing the first kind of registration obtained in the UK, we find that 8 per cent of overseas-qualified hospital doctors were temporarily registered at the beginning, but subsequently acquired full registration. Thus, as shown in Table II.4, 45 per cent were temporarily registered initially, and 37 per cent were temporarily registered at the time of the survey.

The TRAB examination was introduced in 1975. At the time of the survey (September 1977 to February 1978) only 5 per cent of overseas-qualified doctors had taken TRAB, or 17 per cent of the temporarily registered.

As a consequence of the Medical Act 1978, temporary registration has now been replaced by limited registration, the important difference being that doctors having limited registration may qualify for full registration after a period of five years in the United Kingdom.

Geographical distribution
Within each of the fourteen NHS regions, a substantial proportion of hospital doctors were born overseas, according to DHSS statistics[2]. The region with the lowest proportion is South Western (20 per cent) and the one with the highest is North Western (40 per cent). Overseas-born doctors account for at least 28 per cent of all hospital doctors in every region except South Western, Wessex and the notional region comprising the London postgraduate hospitals. Thus, as Appendix Table A5 shows, overseas-born hospital doctors are fairly evenly spread across the country.

---

2 The DHSS statistics are here preferred because the sample for the PSI survey was drawn from 49 Health Districts, which is rather too few to allow reliable analysis by fourteen regions.

In the case of GPs, however, the geographical distribution is more uneven (A 6). Here we have to rely on survey data, and it is necessary to group the regions into pairs in order to produce an adequate base for analysis. The proportion of all GPs who qualified overseas ranges from 3 per cent in Wessex and South Western to 27 per cent in NW and NE Thames, with a number of gradations between. This regional distribution is related to the distribution between conurbation and non-conurbation areas. Overseas-qualified GPs are concentrated within conurbation areas, where 23 per cent of all GPs are overseas-qualified, compared with 11 per cent of GPs elsewhere. Overseas-qualified GPs tend to be concentrated in those regions, and specifically in the conurbations within them, where ethnic minority groups in general also tend to live. One possible reason for this is that overseas-qualified doctors who become GPs in this country have decided to stay more or less permanently, and they tend to choose a practice in an area close to their friends, who will often be members of their own ethnic group. (The same would not apply to hospital doctors, who intend to stay in this country for a limited period, and who tend to move from one post to another at fairly short intervals). However, it may also be the case that practices in the conurbations tend to be less attractive and less in demand than those elsewhere. It may be that overseas-qualified GPs take such practices not from choice but because they find it difficult or impossible to obtain something better.

A different aspect of geographical distribution, which is relevant to hospital doctors although not to GPs, is proximity to an undergraduate teaching hospital. The access which a hospital doctor has to suitable training and educational facilities will depend on what is provided not only within his own hospital but also in the group of hospitals to which it is linked. In the past, the quality of postgraduate training and education available varied widely between different individual hospitals and groups of hospitals. For some time efforts have been made to provide more equal opportunities by improving training arrangements within hospitals and groups of hospitals in which standards of training were previously low. Nevertheless, substantial inequalities still remain. The undergraduate teaching hospitals were traditionally the principal centres of excellence for postgraduate training and education as well as for undergraduate studies. The Health Districts in which they are now located are now designated Teaching Districts. Postgraduate training and educational opportunities in Teaching Districts are generally thought to be superior to those available elsewhere, and jobs in such districts tend to carry more prestige. On the assumption that overseas-qualified and British-qualified doctors have similar training opportunities, we should therefore expect to find that the two groups were distributed across teaching and non-teaching districts in a similar way.

It can be seen from Table II.5 that this is not so. Forty-six per cent of British qualified hospital doctors are working in a teaching district, compared with only 17 per cent of sub-continental and 18 per cent of Arab doctors. It is highly significant that overseas doctors who qualified in a white anglophone country are like British doctors in this respect — 47 per cent of them are working in teaching districts.

Table II.5   Proportion of hospital doctors working in a teaching district, by country of qualification

	Per cent of each group working in a teaching district
All hospital doctors	38
Hospital doctors who first qualified in:	
UK/Eire	46
White anglophone countries	47
Indian sub-continent	17
Arab countries/Iran	18
Elsewhere or country of qualification not known	30

Grade and specialty of hospital doctors

Doctors in hospitals work in teams, and broadly speaking each team consists of a number of junior doctors of various grades working under a single consultant. Where two or more consultants co-operate closely, the team will really consist of several consultants with a common pool of junior doctors, though even then each junior will be formally responsible to one particular consultant. The consultants alone have full responsibility for patients. While junior doctors, particularly those at the higher grades, may in practice do everything that a consultant can do, they are still formally acting under a consultant's instructions. Up to the level of consultant there are five junior grades, but once consultant status is reached (typically after ten to fifteen years in the hospital service) no further promotion is possible, although some consultants may achieve substantial increases in pay through being granted a merit award.

Just over one-third (35 per cent) of all hospital doctors are consultants. If it is borne in mind that medicine is a personal service, that only consultants can take ultimate responsibility for patients and that consultant status is often reached after twelve or thirteen years, this is a very small proportion. If a doctor starts work in the hospital service at 24, he can reasonably expect to reach consultant status by the age of 37, and he will retire at 65. This means that a doctor who achieves consultant status will typically spend 28 years as a consultant having previously spent 13 years as a junior hospital doctor. It is easy to see that if all

15

Table II.6 Grade of hospital doctors, by country of qualification

Column percentages

| | Total | UK/Eire | All overseas | Country of qualification: | | | | |
				White anglo-phone	Indian sub-continent	Arab countries/ Iran	Other overseas	All anglo-phone
House officer	7	10	1	2	1	—	2	1
Senior house officer	26	19	42	20	45	48	37	44
Registrar	19	14	31	29	32	35	24	31
Senior registrar	7	7	7	14	7	6	4	6
Medical assistant[1]	2	1	4	1	4	2	4	4
Consultant	35	45	12	33	9	7	19	10
Not stated	3	2	3	—	3	3	10	4
Base: Hospital doctors								
Unweighted	*1,251*	*539*	*712*	*60*	*454*	*107*	*91*	*652*
Weighted	*2,567*	*1,733*	*834*	*84*	*527*	*115*	*107*	*749*

1 Senior House Medical Officers, of whom the numbers are very small, are grouped with Medical Assistants.

juniors turned into consultants[3], there could only be half as many juniors as consultants at any one time, unless the total number of hospital doctors was constantly and rapidly expanding. In fact, there are twice as many juniors as consultants, and not half as many. This structure is what mainly determines the intake of overseas doctors into the hospital service and their position within it.

The distribution of hospital doctors among the different grades is analysed by country of qualification in Table II.6. Whereas 45 per cent of British-qualified doctors are consultants, only 12 per cent of overseas-qualified doctors have reached this status. White anglophones are again more like British-qualified doctors than like other overseas doctors: 33 per cent of them are consultants. Among overseas-qualified doctors excluding anglophones, only 10 per cent have reached consultant status. In fact, these figures rather understate the extent of the contrast. Partly because of the requirements for temporary registration, overseas doctors tend to migrate well after they have reached the house officer stage; only one per cent of them are at this level, compared with 10 per cent of British-qualified hospital doctors. If we leave this group out of the reckoning and base the calculations on those doctors at senior house officer level or above, we find that 51 per cent of the British-qualified are consultants compared with 10 per cent of the overseas-qualified less anglophones.

We have already seen (p.11) that overseas hospital doctors tend to be in the 35-44 age group and thus at an earlier stage of their careers. Whether their degree of concentration in the junior grades is what would be expected, or whether they have been held back by unequal opportunities is a complex question which will be considered in later chapters. The point that needs to be established here is that the present medical management structure is only possible because there are large numbers of overseas doctors in junior grades, most of whom will leave the country before reaching consultant status or soon after reaching it. Without this constantly renewed pool of junior doctors from abroad, either the period before reaching consultant status would have to be greatly extended, so that doctors would not become consultants, say, until the age of fifty, or the number of consultants relative to the number of juniors would have to be greatly increased on the assumption that the present level of medical care would be maintained (or improved). In detail, this argument has to be modified to take into account the outflow of junior hospital doctors into general practice, academic jobs and so on, but the general form of the reasoning remains valid.

The other main principle of organisation of medical staff in hospitals is by specialty. The division of hospital doctors into the two major groups of surgeons and physicians began early in medical history, and

---

3 In fact, some of the juniors go into general practice or other medical careers, but not enough to affect the general shape of this argument, which is here put in its simplest form.

has been followed in modern times by an accelerating tendency towards further specialisation. Functional specialisation within hospitals is accompanied by the development of corresponding professional organisations. The two oldest and largest Royal Colleges, the Royal College of Surgeons and the Royal College of Physicians, have each recognised an increasing number of sub-specialties, so that doctors in these fields, when they have completed their postgraduate training and examinations, may either be qualified as general physicians or surgeons, or in some more specialised branch. Anaesthetics early became a separate function within hospitals, and later a special faculty of the Royal College of Surgeons was created for anaesthetists, which confers a separate qualification. Groups with clearly defined functions — obstetricians and gynaecologists, pathologists, radiologists, psychiatrists — created entirely separate Royal Colleges. One case which is of particular importance in the context of this inquiry is geriatrics. The treatment of old patients in hospitals is not necessarily a separate function, since most of the illnesses of the old have much in common with the illnesses of younger people, and patients need not necessarily be segregated according to their age. However, various pressures have led to an increasing functional separation of this kind, while geriatricians have remained within the Royal College of Physicians.

At the early stages of his career a young doctor needs to obtain experience of a number of different specialties, but well before he is ready to become a consultant, he should have gravitated to the specialty in which he will finally make his career. An outstanding problem of medical manpower planning is that some specialties are more popular than others. The Department of Health and Social Security uses a number of indicators of the balance between supply and demand of doctors within each specialty, and these show very wide variations. An alternative measure is available from within the survey. These measures show, for example, that general medicine and general surgery are among the most popular specialties, while geriatrics is among the least popular.

Table II.7 compares the distribution across specialties of British-qualified and overseas-qualified doctors. Overseas doctors tend very strongly to be concentrated in geriatrics, and to a lesser extent in orthopaedics, anaesthetics and surgical specialties other than general surgery. They are under-represented in general medicine, in other medical specialties apart from geriatrics, in general surgery, radiology and radiotherapy and pathology. This pattern seems broadly consistent with the theory that overseas doctors have difficulty in getting jobs in the more popular specialties and therefore tend to be channelled into the less popular ones. This question will be analysed in detail in a later chapter.

Postgraduate medical qualifications
The qualification that is now generally expected of applicants for consultant posts is membership or fellowship of a British Royal College. The

Table II.7 Specialty of British and overseas-qualified hospital doctors

Column percentages

	Country of qualification	
	UK/Eire	Overseas
Paediatrics	5	3
Geriatrics	2	9
General Medicine	14	7
Other medical specialties	6	4
All medical specialties less geriatrics	*25*	*14*
All medical specialties	*27*	*24*
Orthopaedics	5	9
General Surgery	11	9
Other surgical specialties	5	8
All surgical specialties	*20*	*26*
Anaesthetics	9	12
Radiology/radiotherapy	7	4
Gynaecology/obstetrics	8	9
All pathology specialties	8	4
All psychiatric specialties	8	10
Accident and emergency	3	3
Other specialties	6	5
Not stated	4	3
Base: Hospital doctors		
Unweighted	*539*	*712*
Weighted	*1,733*	*834*

See Appendix B for an explanation of this grouping of specialties.

Royal Colleges award membership (or fellowship in the case of the Royal College of Surgeons) to those who have passed an examination in two or more parts. The various parts of these examinations cover the ability to deal with clinical or practical problems (in the great majority of specialties where this is appropriate) as well as theoretical knowledge. Doctors are not eligible to take these examinations until they have worked for specified periods in specified types of job; by deciding which posts to recognise for this purpose, the Royal Colleges can exercise some control over the quality of training received by doctors before they are allowed to become examination candidates. The amount of control that they actually exercise in this way varies widely: the requirements may be highly specific or fairly vague.

A second broad group of qualifications is diplomas in specialist subjects granted by Royal Colleges, by conjoint boards in which more than one Royal College is involved and by universities. These are less advanced qualifications than the membership or fellowship, although the value and content varies widely between different diplomas.

19

A third broad group is the academic postgraduate medical qualifications, such as the Doctor of Medicine (MD) and Master of Surgery (MS) which are intended for those who are pursuing a career in research or teaching.

We shall consistently use the hierarchical form of analysis of postgraduate medical qualifications that is shown in Table II.8. The qualifications are taken in the order shown, and doctors are classified according to the highest qualification on the list that they have. The table shows that British hospital doctors are substantially better qualified than overseas hospital doctors, if fellowship or membership of a Royal College is taken as the main criterion: 52 per cent of British hospital doctors compared with 26 per cent of overseas hospital doctors have membership or fellowship. However, overseas hospital doctors are more likely than British ones to have one of the lower qualifications, and the proportions of the two groups having no postgraduate qualification are fairly similar (31 per cent of British hospital doctors compared with 38 per cent of overseas hospital doctors). The difference between the two groups is the one that would be expected from the fact that overseas doctors are mostly in the younger age groups, more junior, and at an earlier stage of their careers in this country.

Table II.8 Highest postgraduate medical qualification, by type of job and country of first qualification

Column percentages

	GPs		Hospital Doctors	
	British-qualified	Overseas-qualified	British-qualified	Overseas-qualified
Membership or Fellowship of a British Royal College	7	18	52	26
Membership or Fellowship of a British Royal College, Part 1 only	4	4	7	14
British Diploma	35	26	6	9
British MD/MS/MSc	1	—	1	—
Membership or Fellowship of a foreign college/foreign diploma	1	4	*	8
Foreign MD/MS/MSc	—	2	—	4
ECFMG[1]	*	1	3	2
None of these/not stated	52	45	31	38
Base: All informants				
Unweighted	*477*	*253*	*539*	*712*
Weighted	*1,649*	*274*	*1,733*	*834*

1 Education Commission Foreign Medical Graduates (USA).

However, overseas doctors who have become GPs tend to have better postgraduate qualifications than British GPs as Table II.8 shows. The overseas-qualified are more likely to have the membership or fellowship (18 per cent compared with 7 per cent), and while a higher proportion of the British than of the overseas GPs have a British diploma, this difference is offset by the foreign qualifications held by the overseas GPs. This finding suggests (as further analyses will confirm) that a relatively high proportion of overseas-qualified GPs have gone into general practice late after taking membership or fellowship examinations and after trying to pursue a specialist career.

III Command of English

Overseas-qualified doctors tend to work in hospitals rather than in general practice; within the hospital service they are heavily concentrated in the more junior grades, and to a lesser extent, within the less popular specialties. Before analysing these differences further in order to show how far they arise from unequal opportunities, it is important to find a way of assessing the effect of language competence. The great majority of overseas-qualified doctors are not native English speakers. Clearly, their career progress, and the benefit that they derive from experience and training within the NHS, may depend to a considerable extent on their command of English. Of course, command of English is not a simple attribute that can be exhaustively described by defining a position on a scale from good to bad. There is a wide range of relevant language skills. In particular, doctors need to have some command of contrasting styles of speech that are appropriate to different contexts, for example, the technical language used in medical discussion and literature, the colloquial, middle-class English used among doctors on less formal occasions, and the local, colloquial English used by patients. To the extent that the command of these different styles of speech can be reduced to a single score, there is still the question as to what level of skill, or what score, is high enough to allow a doctor to practice satisfactorily, or to be at no significant disadvantage compared with native English speakers.

Description of the English language test
A special test of command of styles of English relevant to doctors was devised for this study. All survey informants were asked to complete this test, and 95 per cent of them agreed to do so. Informants can, therefore, be classified according to their language test scores. This makes possible two kinds of analysis. First, the experience of high and low scoring overseas-qualified doctors can be compared. If the experience of the two groups is similar, then it follows that inadequate command of English is unlikely to be the prime cause of disadvantages suffered by either group. Secondly, we can identify a group of overseas-qualified doctors who score as high, or nearly as high, as British-qualified doctors. To the extent that these high scoring overseas doctors encounter greater dif-

ficulties than British doctors in making a career within the NHS, we can conclude that these difficulties do not arise principally from a difference in their command of English.

These kinds of analysis will only be useful to the extent that the test is a reliable and valid measure of the relevant language skills. It is, therefore, worth describing the test in some detail and referring to the evidence as to its reliability and validity. The test consisted of thirty items in three groups of ten items each. The first group of items were nouns or noun phrases used in common speech for which there is an exactly equivalent medical term. In each case, the interviewer read out the common term, while the informant was asked to pick out the corresponding medical term from a list of four possibilities. For example:

Thrush   nephritis
                  diabetes mellitus
                  tinea circinata
                  monilia

(The correct answer is monilia.) This simultaneously tests understanding of the common and of the medical term.

The second group of items were colloquial or slangy phrases that patients are likely to use in the consulting room; some of them describe medical conditions, some deal euphemistically or crudely with sexual functions, and some express very basic ideas (such as being tired) which regularly occur in a medical context. Again, the interviewer read out the phrase, while the informant picked out the equivalent phrase in completely plain English from a list of four. For example:

I am whacked   I am exhausted
                  I have been beaten
                  I am feeling elated
                  I have lost all my money

It will be noticed that some of the wrong answers are plausible to someone who does not have a complete command of English idiom.

For each of the first two groups of items, the informant played a passive role; that is, he was not required to produce his own words, nor to manipulate words given to him, but only to pick out an equivalent word or phrase. For the third group of items, however, the informant played an active role. These items were based on common verbs which are used with prepositions, such as 'looking forward to'. The informant was given a list of sentences like the following one:

My car has stopped working (BREAK)

The informant was then asked to produce an equivalent sentence, using the verb shown in brackets after the sentence together with a preposition:

My car has broken down.

This group of items tests the ability to use some very common expressions which often give difficulty to people whose first language is not

23

English. In order to give a correct answer, the informant has to find the appropriate preposition, and to manipulate the word order and the tense of the verb correctly. Most, but not all, of these items related closely or loosely to a medical context.

Validation of the test
The first step in analysis of this test was to consider the responses to individual items. For 28 of the 30 items, at least 88 percent of British-qualified doctors gave the correct response, and for 21 items at least 95 per cent answered correctly. The two items which less than the great majority of British-qualified doctors answered correctly were 'acid head' (taker of LSD) (50 per cent) and 'pretends' (= makes out that) (67 per cent). It was decided not to include 'acid head' in the final test score, because too few native English speakers understood the term, and also because it correlated relatively weakly with the other items. 'Makes out that' was retained.

The proportions of overseas-qualified doctors who answered correctly were generally markedly lower, although the difference between British and overseas-qualified doctors varied widely between items (Table A 7). This simply implies that some of the items are much harder than others for people who are not native English speakers. The harder items, which produce larger differences between the two groups, could be said to be better discriminators than the easier ones, and on this ground it could be argued that the easier items ought to be discarded. However, we did not take this view, because we wanted the overall test score to reflect the informant's ability to cope with a range of linguistic tasks.

The next step in the analysis was to assign an overall score to each informant on the basis of the number of items that he had correctly answered by assigning one point for each correct answer. Statistical tests established that responses to each individual item, with the exception of 'acid head', correlated strongly with responses to all of the others. From this, and from a split-half reliability test, it was established that the overall test score had good reliability (see Appendix B).

It is relatively easy to establish the reliability of a test (roughly speaking, its stability), but far more difficult to show that it is valid (roughly speaking, that it measures what it purports to measure). In this case there are three independent checks on validity:

(a)   The actual content of the items can be inspected.
(b)   The test score can be related to the linguistic background of the informant. Those whose native language is English would be expected to score much higher than others, and to the extent that they do, this tends to show that the test is valid.
(c)   At the end of the survey interview, interviewers rated the informant's command of English using four-point scales on four dimensions: (i) accent, (ii) how easily the interviewer understood the informant, (iii) how easily the informant understood the interviewer, and (iv)

an overall rating.[1] These interviewer ratings can be related to the overall test score, and the stronger this relationship is found to be the more confident we can be in the validity of the test.

As regards the actual content of the items, the general description already given is enough to establish, prima facie, that the test measures relevant language skills. In terms of subject matter the test covers:

diseases
parts of the body
mental and physical states
sexual functions
drugs and alcohol (although the item on drugs had to be
   dropped)
behaviour and activities.

In terms of styles of speech, the test covers technical medical language, standard colloquial idiom and slangy or crude colloquialisms. It tests both comprehension and the use of language. There can, of course, be endless discussion about the merits of particular items. For example, it may be said that certain items are old-fashioned or upper-middle class ('the curse' to mean menstruation may fall into this category) and that others are regional (such as 'tight' to mean slightly drunk), but over the thirty items there is a reasonable balance between different styles of English used in different contexts by different sorts of people.

The most powerful evidence of the validity of the test comes from relating the scores to the linguistic background of the informant. It was established from the interview whether the informant spoke English at home as a child, and if so, whether English was his only childhood language, and whether he received his schooling and medical education entirely or mainly in English. From this, informants can be classified into the six groups shown in Table III.1, running from those who spoke only English at home as a child to those who neither spoke English at home as a child nor were taught in English at either school or medical college. (Informants are classified according to the earliest context in which they used English.)

The great majority of British qualified doctors (90 per cent) spoke English at home as children, (the remainder are mostly doctors who grew up overseas but qualified in Britain). A substantial proportion of overseas-qualified doctors (30 per cent) spoke English at home as children, and a further 54 per cent were taught in English both at school and at medical college. Only 5 per cent used English in none of the three contexts. Thus, very few overseas-qualified doctors are people who had little or no experience of using English before they came to Britain. Because medical education is conducted in English in most of the countries from which they come, most overseas-qualified doctors at least

---

1 These interviewer ratings were recorded *before* the informant completed the language test.

studied medicine in English, if they had not previously used it at school or in the home. For this reason their command of colloquial or idiomatic English is more likely to be limited than their command of technical or medical language: it is therefore the idiomatic usages with which the test is mostly concerned.

**Table III.1 Earliest context in which English was used,
by country of first qualification**

Column percentages

	Country of first qualification:	
	UK/Eire	Elsewhere
Only English spoken at home in childhood	87 ⎤	13 ⎤
English and other language(s) spoken	⎟ 90	⎟ 30
at home in childhood	4 ⎦	17 ⎦
English used at school *and* at medical college	1	54
English used at medical college but not at school	9	6
English used at school but not at medical college	—	4
English *not* spoken in childhood at home, nor used at school nor at medical college	—	5
Base: All informants		
Unweighted	*1,016*	*965*
Weighted	*3,382*	*1,108*

Table A8 shows that there are very strong relationships between the test score and the informant's linguistic background (among overseas-qualified doctors alone.) Those whose only language as a child was English score very much higher than the rest, and generally speaking it is true that the earlier the context in which an informant used English the higher he will tend to score. However, it is interesting that those who used English in none of the three contexts — home, school, or medical college — score, if anything, rather higher than those who used English either at school or at college (but not in both contexts). It may be that these doctors, who came to Britain without much previous experience of using English, were more conscious of their lack of English than those who had some little previous experience and were, therefore, more likely to make special efforts to catch up.

The third method of checking the validity of the test is by relating the test score to the interviewer's rating made at the end of the interview. Table III.2 groups overseas-qualified doctors according to their test scores, and shows for each group the proportion who were given the highest rating on each of the four aspects of command of English which were rated. For each of the four ratings the relationships are extremely strong.

If the overall rating is taken as an example, it shows that 76 per cent of overseas-qualified doctors with maximum or nearly maximum test scores (28 or 29) were rated as having 'perfect' English, compared with 4 per cent of those having test scores from 0 to 14. As might be expected, informants' accents are rated lower than their comprehension or comprehensibility. Informants could understand rather more easily than they were understood.

Table III.2 **Interviewer's assessment of informant's English, by language test score: overseas-qualified doctors**

Percentages

Four separate interviewer ratings	Language test score:					
	0-14	15-18	19-23	24-25	26-27	28-29
Little or no accent	2	4	14	19	27	55
Very easy to understand	7	25	40	53	63	85
Informant understands very easily	11	25	48	58	71	93
Overall assessment — perfect	4	9	23	33	46	76
Base: Overseas-qualified doctors						
Unweighted	*123*	*161*	*289*	*126*	*119*	*94*
Weighted	*135*	*181*	*333*	*143*	*132*	*113*

NB: Assessments were four-point rating scales; only the highest point on each scale is shown in this table.

Command of English as measured by the test

It is difficult to say what level of language skill, or exactly what test score, is high enough to allow a doctor to practise satisfactorily. However, some light can be thrown on the question by the relationships between test scores and interviewers' ratings. It seems from these analyses that only those scoring 0-18 have a significant linguistic handicap, because it is only among this group that a significant proportion are considered by the interviewers to have English that is not perfect or good: 39 per cent of those scoring 0-14 and 25 per cent of those scoring 15-18, or 31 per cent of the two groups combined are considered to have poor English.

On this interpretation, about two-thirds of overseas-qualified doctors (excluding those from white anglophone countries) have no significant linguistic handicap, while 31 per cent (who score between 0-18) probably have some handicap, although it may be slight in many cases. This latter group is made up of 18 per cent who score between 15-18 (more than half of the items correctly answered) and only 13 per cent who score less than 15 (less than half of the items correctly answered). It is probably mainly among this latter 13 per cent that there are doctors with more than a slight linguistic handicap.

Table III.3 Interviewer's overall assessment of informant's English, by language test score: overseas-qualified doctors

Column percentages

Assessment of informant's overall English ability	Language test score:					
	0-14	15-18	19-23	24-25	26-27	28-29
Perfect	4	9	23	33	46	76
Good	58	65	66	61	50	24
Rather poor	38	24	9	3	—	—
Very poor	1	1	—	—	—	—
Not stated	—	2	2	3	5	—
Base: Overseas-qualified doctors						
Unweighted	*123*	*161*	*289*	*126*	*119*	*94*
Weighted	*135*	*181*	*333*	*143*	*132*	*113*

GPs tend to score higher than hospital doctors: only 12 per cent of overseas-qualified GPs (excluding white anglophones) score 0-18, compared with 38 per cent of hospital doctors. The reason for this is that overseas-qualified GPs tend to be older and to have lived in Britain for longer than overseas-qualified hospital doctors. Separate analyses clearly show, as might be expected, that those who have been in Britain for longer tend to achieve higher language test scores.

Analysis by country of origin in detail (Table A9) shows that doctors from Arab countries score lowest. This is because a significant proportion of Arabs, unlike Indians, did not receive their medical education in

Table III.4 Language test score, by type of job: overseas-qualified doctors excluding white anglophones

	Total	GPs	Hospital doctors
0-14[1]	13 ⎤ 31	3 ⎤ 12	17 ⎤ 38
15-18[1]	18 ⎦	9 ⎦	21 ⎦
19-23	32	30	33
24-25	12	17	11
26-27	11	19	8
28-29	6	13	4
Test not done	7	8	6

[1] Groups within which a significant proportion of informants are judged to have some linguistic handicap.

English, and also because Arab doctors tend to have arrived in Britain recently.

It is doctors at the lower grades in the hospital service who are most likely to have inadequate English (Table A10). Among overseas-qualified hospital doctors, 50 per cent of those at house officer or senior house officer level score 0-14, compared with 32 per cent of registrars, 9 per cent of senior registrars and 7 per cent of consultants. Thus, there is no significant language problem among senior registrars and above.

IV Expectations and Experience of Migrants

This chapter describes the migration of overseas doctors to the UK from their own point of view. It looks in some detail at the migrants' expectations on coming to this country in the light of their subsequent experience, as they see it. Here there are no comparisons with British doctors, because we are reconstructing the migrants' perspective. Objective comparisons between the career progress and present experience of British and indigenous doctors are made in subsequent chapters, which aim to show how far the views of overseas doctors about their experience in Britain are justified by the facts.

Timing of the migration

Of our population of doctors in the NHS in England, 31 per cent were born outside the United Kingdom. Of these overseas-born doctors, half (49 per cent) came to the UK from 1970 onwards, about one-quarter (27 per cent) came in the 1960s, and about one-quarter (23 per cent) before

Table IV.1 **Year of first coming to the UK, by type of job: doctors born outside the United Kingdom.**

Column percentages

Year of first coming to the UK	Total	General practitioners	Hospital doctors
Up to 1959	23	44	15
1960-1969	27	45	20
1970-1974	28 ⎤ 49	10 ⎤ 10	34 ⎤ 63
1975-1978	21 ⎦	— ⎦	29 ⎦
Not stated	1	1	1

Base: Doctors born outside the United Kingdom			
Unweighted	1,169	359	810
Weighted	1,371	391	981

Q4 Not counting short visits of less than 6 months, in what month and year did you first come to Britain?

1960. It follows that among overseas-born doctors who are now in this country, the numbers who came in any particular year decrease as we move backwards in time. The principal reason for this is, of course, that many migrants leave the country again after a period, so that comparatively few remain from earlier years. It may also be the case that for years before 1960 the numbers coming into the country were lower than subsequently.

Doctors from Arab countries and Iran tend to be the most recent migrants (Table A11) probably because of a recent increase in the inflow from these areas. Doctors from continental Europe tend to be the earliest migrants (54 per cent came to the UK before 1950). Many of these people were political refugees, and do not essentially form a part of the migration for medical training and experience with which we are mainly concerned; also, many obtained their primary medical qualification in Britain.

There is a strong tendency for overseas-born GPs to be earlier migrants than overseas-born hospital doctors, because nearly all migrants come to train and work in the hospital service. Among those who have stayed, some have become GPs after a period in the hospital service.

When overseas-born doctors first came to the UK, they were typically aged between 25 and 30; 49 per cent were within this age range at the time of migration, and therefore probably migrated within a few years of qualifying as a doctor. One-quarter migrated at a later age than this, and one-quarter at an earlier age: most of the latter group are overseas-born, but British-qualified. Those born in the Indian sub-continent or an Arab country are particularly likely to have migrated when aged 25-30, whereas those born in continental Europe, a white anglophone country or elsewhere are more likely to have migrated at an earlier age (Table A12). A significant part of the migration from these latter three areas was probably unconnected with medical training or career considerations, but was rather a response to political or family circumstances.

This analysis can be reinforced by considering the stage in their education or career at which the migrants came to the UK (Table IV.2). Among those born and qualified overseas, 7 per cent came immediately after completing the Bachelor of Medicine degree (MB), 20 per cent within two years of completing it, and the remaining 73 per cent at some later stage. However, among all those born outside the UK (regardless of their country of qualification), there are 15 per cent who came to this country at some time before completing secondary school, and a further 5 per cent who came at the start of or during undergraduate medical education. When considering the decision to come to the UK, and migrants' expectations compared with their subsequent experience, we shall confine our attention to those who came at the start of undergraduate medical education or at some later stage. This group, referred to as 'adult migrants', accounts for 85 per cent of all doctors born overseas.

Table IV.2 Stage of coming to the UK. (Q6)

Column percentages

Stage of coming to the UK	Doctors born outside the United Kingdom	Doctors born and qualified overseas
Up to the end of primary school	9	*
After primary school, before completing secondary school	6	*
At the start of undergraduate medical education	4	*
During undergraduate medical education	1	*
Immediately after completing the MB or its equivalent	6	7
Up to 2 years after completing the MB or its equivalent	16	20
More than 2 years after completing the MB or its equivalent	58	73
Unweighted	*1,169*	*958*
Weighted	*1,371*	*1,094*

NB Informants in last five groups are referred to as 'adult migrants'.

Separation of families

About half of the adult migrants were already married when they came to the UK and just under one-third had children at that time. Generally speaking, the migration has not led to the separation of families for long periods, although there was some tendency for doctors to come to the UK without their families at first, and for their families to join them later. Only four per cent of migrants are currently separated from their wives or husbands, who have remained in the home country; and while 62 per cent now have children, only six per cent are separated from them. Fuller details are shown in Table IV.3.

Country of origin of wife or husband

Confining our attention to adult migrants who are now married, and excluding white anglophones and doctors who qualified in the UK, we find that among the men, 17 per cent are married to a British person and 75 per cent to someone from the country of origin (the remainder are married to someone from neither Britain nor the country of origin). About two-thirds of this group were already married before they came to this country, while about one-third have got married since coming, and have therefore had the opportunity to marry a British person; 17 per cent (or about half of those who have had the opportunity) have done so. Thus,

Table IV.3 Migration of wife or husband and children by sex

			Percentages
	Total	Men	Women
Not married on arrival in UK	48	48	50
Married on arrival:			
Spouse came with informant	18	17	26
Spouse already in the UK	2	1	9
Spouse came later, within less than 1 year	19	22	7
Spouse came 1 year or more later	8	9	1
Spouse has not yet come	4	3	7
Not married or had no children on arrival in UK	69	67	77
Married with child(ren) on arrival:			
All children came with informant	15	16	13
Some children came with informant	1	1	1
No children came with informant	15	16	10
Not now married	21	18	39
Now married, no child(ren) aged under 16	17	17	16
Now married with child(ren) aged under 16:			
All children now in UK	56	59	39
Some or all children now outside UK	6	6	5
Base: Adult migrants			
Unweighted	*1,016*	*852*	*164*
Weighted	*1,160*	*972*	*188*

an important minority of the male migrants now have close family ties with this country.

Among the women migrants, the picture is completely different. Only 4 per cent are married to a British person, while 89 per cent are married to someone from the country of origin. This follows a pattern that has been observed in other groups of migrants. Men are generally more likely than women to inter-marry with the host population, probably because they are more likely to play an outgoing social role.

Information, finance, finding a job
Adult migrants were asked the forcing question 'From what source or sources did you obtain information about medical training or careers in Britain before you came?'. This question makes it difficult for an informant to admit that he had no reliable source of information. Even so, a

comparatively small proportion of adult migrants said that they had obtained information from an authoritative British or foreign body (Table A13). Only 28 per cent mentioned any of the following six official British bodies: the General Medical Council, the British Medical Association, the British Embassy, Consul or High Commission, the Department of Health and Social Security, the Council for Post Graduate Medical Education, a Royal College. Only 32 per cent mentioned any kind of British body or organisation. Eleven per cent mentioned a foreign body, and only 40 per cent mentioned any kind of organisation, whether British or foreign. The remainder seem to have had information only from other doctors or students (28 per cent) or from friends or relatives.

Recent migrants (those who came from 1970 onwards) seem to have had rather more reliable information, in that a higher proportion mentioned one of the six main British bodies (32 per cent, compared with 22 per cent of earlier migrants). However, this only fractionally modifies the general picture, which is that a majority of overseas doctors came to the UK without first obtaining reliable information about medical training and careers in this country from an authoritative British body. In these circumstances, it would not be surprising to find that their expectations had not been adjusted to reality and that they had little prior knowledge of the problems they were likely to encounter in pursuing a medical career in this country. The Council for Post Graduate Medical Education now acts as the focal point for enquiries about careers and training in the UK, but the evidence is that it reaches only a small minority of migrants; only two per cent of those who came to the UK from 1970 onwards mentioned the Council.

The great majority of adult migrants (94 per cent) had already qualified as doctors before they came here, and most of these expected to practise in this country immediately. Of those who were qualified when they came, 25 per cent had obtained a medical job in the UK before coming, 36 per cent found one within four weeks, and a further 10 per cent in five to eight weeks. Apart from the 4 per cent for whom we have no information, this leaves 25 per cent who clearly had difficulty in finding a job within a reasonable time. Among these, 5 per cent took 31 weeks or more to find a job (among whom 3 per cent took a year or more), 9 per cent took 17 to 30 weeks, and 11 per cent took 9 to 16 weeks. In short, three quarters of migrants came to this country first and looked for a job when they got here, in most cases having no reliable prior information as to whether the kind of job that they wanted was available. Among these are 46 per cent who had found a medical job (not necessarily the kind that they ideally wanted) within eight weeks and 25 per cent who we know had difficulties, leading in a substantial minority of cases to a lengthy period of unemployment.[1]

---

1 Where a doctor, for example, took a holiday on arrival, the time taken to find a job is counted from the time when he started to look for one.

Reasons for migrating

A first approach to an understanding of doctors' reasons for migrating is to consider their answers to the straightforward open quesion 'Why did you come to Britain?'. This question is open in the sense that doctors' answers were recorded in their own words and classified afterwards, and also in the sense that it gives no clues as to the kind of answer that is expected. In particular, informants are free to mention reasons to do with the advantages of life in this country and to do with the disadvantages of life in the country of origin and they can emphasise their career and training or other factors.

Table IV.4 Reasons for coming to the UK

	Per cent
Career/training	
To obtain further cualifications/for postgraduate study	70
To gain more/broader/more up-to-date medical experience	12
Training/facilities/knowledge of newest techniques are better in UK	9
British postgraduate qualifications are (very) highly regarded/superior to local qualifications	4
To advance in the profession/improve myself	4
Suitable training jobs are in short supply in country of origin/not possible to train in country of origin	2
Better pay/standard of living in UK	1
Better working conditions in UK	*
Unrelated to career or training	
To see the (western) world, travel, broaden horizons, learn a new language	12
Political or religious difficulties in country of origin	6
To join spouse or children	5
Already had friends or relatives in UK	4
Long-standing links with UK, e.g. wartime service	3
Advice from friends or relatives/family tradition	2
Other answers	3
Base: Adult migrants	
Unweighted	*1,016*
Weighted	*1,160*

Q9 Why did you come to Britain?

The great majority of adult migrants (70 per cent) said that they came to the UK to obtain further qualifications or for postgraduate study.

Most of the other answers connected with careers and training were essentially similar, although with a different emphasis. Thus, 12 per cent of adult migrants emphasised broader or more up-to-date medical experience, 9 per cent particularly mentioned the use of newest techniques in the UK and 4 per cent mentioned the superiority of British postgraduate qualifications. All of these answers carry the implication that the doctor intended to leave this country after a period. Very small proportions of migrants gave career-based answers that seem to carry the opposite implication. Thus, only four per cent said that they had come here to advance in the profession or to improve themselves (the common attitude of the permanent immigrant) while only one per cent mentioned a better standard of living or working conditions available in the UK. The great majority of career-based answers are expressed as specific advantages of working and training in the UK for a limited period and not as disadvantages of remaining in the country of origin. Only two per cent of migrants said they had come to this country because it was not possible to train in the country of origin.

A significant minority of migrants gave answers unrelated to careers or training. Twelve per cent said they had migrated to see the world, to broaden their horizons, and so on, 5 per cent to join their wives, husbands or children, and 4 per cent to join other relatives or friends who were already in the UK. There is a small group (6 per cent) who left the home country to escape from political or religious difficulties.

While this open question provides a good conspectus of doctors' reasons for migrating, the relative importance of more precisely defined reasons can be explored through the answers to further, more specific questions. The answers to the open question suggest that reasons connected with careers and training were much the most important for the majority of informants. This was confirmed when informants were asked 'Did you come to Britain chiefly in order to further your medical training or career or chiefly for other reasons?'. Of all adult migrants, 85 per cent said they had come chiefly to further their medical training or careers, but there are some significant differences between groups. Doctors from the Indian sub-continent and from Arab countries are the most likely to have migrated for career or training reasons (91 per cent and 90 per cent respectively), while those from white anglophone countries are the least likely (62 per cent). Detailed analysis of the open question shows that a substantial proportion of the white anglophones (30 per cent) — more than of any other group — came 'to see the world' or, in other words, as part of the grand European tour that is popular for example among young Australians and New Zealanders.

Earlier migrants (who have stayed) are less likely to have come for career reasons than recent migrants. One reason for this is that among those who came up to 1959 is a significant minority (16 per cent) who were refugees, mostly from Europe. The proportion who came to the UK to escape political or religious persecution is much smaller among more recent migrants. Another reason for the difference is that where doctors came for career or training reasons they usually intended to leave after a period, but where they came for any other reason they were clearly more likely to be making a permanent move.

Table IV.5 Proportion of adult migrants who came to the UK chiefly to further their medical training or career

	Per cent
All adult migrants	**85**
Country of first qualification	
UK/Eire	80
White anglophone country	62
Indian sub-continent	91
Arab country	90
Elsewhere	71
Present post	
GP	78
Hospital doctor	88
Sex	
Male	89
Female	68
Age	
Up to 29	86
30-34	88
35-44	90
45-54	84
55 or over	50
Year of coming to the UK	
Up to 1959	71
1960-64	86
1965-69	89
1970-72	82
1973-74	85
1975-76	90
1977-78	97

Q10 Did you come to Britain chiefly to further your medical training or chiefly for other reasons?

Women are less likely than men to have come to the UK for reasons connected with their own careers (68 per cent compared with 89 per cent). This is because a comparatively high proportion of women (28 per cent) came with their husbands or to join husbands already here. Nevertheless, this difference is not particularly strong, and what perhaps needs to be emphasised is that two-thirds of women migrants did come to the UK for reasons connected with their own careers.

Table IV.6   **Importance of various objectives in coming to the UK (Q12)**

	Per cent of adult migrants who rate each objective as:	
	Very important	Very or quite important
To get a job with better training opportunities	52	77
To obtain a specific kind of training not easily available in country of origin	44	68
To progress faster in the medical profession	35	68
To get medical experience not easily available in country of origin	29	60
To broaden horizons by travel	24	66
For personal reasons	16	32
To escape from political or religious difficulties in country of origin	7	14
To make a fresh start in a country thought to be preferable	6	16
To improve standard of living	5	18

NB Every percentage in this table is based on all adult migrants. The base figure is 1,016 (unweighted) or 1,160 (weighted).

Both the results of the open and of the specific question clearly establish that the majority of migrants came to the UK for reasons connected with their careers or training. An indication of the relative importance of more closely defined career or training objectives is given by the answers to a further question which asked doctors to rate the importance of a series of nine reasons for coming to the UK. The four career-related reasons are rated as more important than any of the five that are unrelated to careers. They are: to get a job with better training opportunities; to obtain a specific kind of training not easily available in the country of origin; to progress faster in the medical profession; to get medical experience not easily available in the country of origin. Most migrants attach considerable importance to all of these four objectives, but the first two are particularly emphasised. The ratings of the five objectives that are unrelated to careers are much what would be expected from answers to previous questions, except that informants attach more importance to 'broadening horizons by travel' when directly asked about it than they do when giving the chief reason for migrating. Detailed analysis reinforces the earlier conclusions that white anglophones attach a higher value than other groups to travel for its own sake, that earlier migrants (and hence those who are now over fifty) are more likely than other groups to have come to the UK to escape from political or religious persecution, and that women are more likely than men to have come to be with their family.

We have seen that the reason for migrating, when related to careers, is usually expressed positively, in terms of the benefits to be had from coming to this country, rather than negatively, in terms of the difficulties encountered in the country of origin. The importance attached to these two sides of the same coin was explored by asking migrants what advantages they hoped to get from coming to the UK to train or pursue a medical career, and also whether they had encountered difficulties in training or pursuing a career in the country of origin, and if so, what difficulties.

Table IV.7   Career or training difficulties in country of origin[1]

	Per cent
Experienced difficulties in career/training	34
Difficulties experienced	
No medical schools/no proper training available/no postgraduate examination system	13
Limited number of places in postgraduate training courses	8
Postgraduate training and examination system not fully developed or well organized	3
Not paid to do a job while training	2
Training/qualifications/experience only available up to a certain level	1
Competitive/had to work	1
Needed to have experience overseas before becoming a senior doctor or consultant	*
Political difficulties/Communism/Nazism trouble in East Africa/expelled/ persecuted	4
Other difficulties	3

1 See note to Table IV.6

Q13 Were there any particular difficulties in pursuing a medical career or getting medical training in your country of origin?
Q14 *If yes* What difficulties?

The question about the advantages of coming to this country merely confirms that nearly all migrants saw the positive benefits that have already been described. On the negative side, we find that one-third of migrants encountered career or training difficulties in the country of origin; the difficulty most often mentioned was the lack of a developed postgraduate training or examination system. A small proportion of migrants mentioned that in the country of origin they could not be paid to do a job and train at the same time; in a number of countries a young doctor needs to get a grant or government support in order to study for further qualifications, whereas in the UK young doctors learn on the job.

Doctors from white anglophone countries were the least likely to have experienced difficulties at home, whereas doctors from Arab countries and those who came to the UK before taking their basic medical qualifications were the most likely to have encountered difficulties. Men were substantially more likely than women to have encountered difficulties in the country of origin (37 per cent compared with 19 per cent). Although a proportion of women came to this country to be with their husbands (and not, therefore, to escape from difficulties at home) this is not enough to explain the difference. There is some suggestion here that women migrants, compared with men, are more likely to be taking advantage of opportunities abroad in an enterprising way rather than avoiding difficulties in pursuing a career in the home country.

Table IV.8 **Proportion of adult migrants who experienced career or training difficulties in country of origin by country of qualification, sex and year of coming to the UK**

	Per cent
Country of qualification	
UK/Eire	48
White anglophone country	16
Indian sub-continent	32
Arab country	45
Elsewhere	42
Sex:	
Male	37
Female	19
Year of coming to the UK	
Up to 1959	41
1960-64	37
1965-69	34
1970-72	30
1973-74	34
1975-76	32
1977-78	35

General Expectations and Experience

A central objective of this study is to establish how far overseas doctors' experience in the NHS, as they see it, has lived up to their expectations.

This can be explored in a broad and general way through the answers to the following series of questions.

Q26 Is there anything about studying or working in Britain that has disappointed you?
Q27 *If yes* What has disappointed you? What else has disappointed you?
Q28 Is there anything about studying or working in Britain that is better than you expected?
Q29 *If yes* What is better than you expected? What else?

Of all adult migrants, 58 per cent said they had some cause for disappointment, and 55 per cent said that some thing or things were better than they had expected. Because there is considerable overlap between these two groups, it is not the case that roughly half of migrants are disappointed and the other half pleased to find that their expectations have been exceeded. In fact, more than one-third of migrants (35 per cent) had mixed feelings; they found some aspects of their experience in this country disappointing, but also found that some things were better than they had expected. Also, exactly one-fifth of migrants found that their expectations were entirely confirmed, and considered that nothing was either better or worse than they had expected. This rather complex picture contains brightness and gloom in about equal proportions, but certainly it is clear that disappointment with at least some aspects of studying and working in the UK is very common.

Table IV.9   Sources of disappointment with studying or working in the UK[1] (Q27)

	Percentage
No disappointment	41
Disappointed with job opportunities:	
Could not get the job I wanted/many applications without success	13
Could not get a good training job in a better hospital, or a job in which I would be able to study	9
Total unable to get suitable job	**21**
Biassed selection from job applicants	3
Colour discrimination in selection or promotion	3
Bias or discrimination	**6**
Frequent job changes	3
Forced to abandon chosen specialty or field	2
Need a particular sequence of jobs which unable to get	1
Any mention of job opportunities	**30**

Table IV.9 (cont'd)

	Percentage
Disappointed with study and training:	
Lack of time for study	9
Inadequate training arrangements or teaching facilities	9
Too little contact teaching/do not see consultant(s) enough	4
Too little medical experience of the kind required	2
Examination system	2
No opportunity to attend courses/criticism of courses	1
Any study or training difficulties	**22**
Disappointed with pay and hours:	
Pay not high enough	5
Pay structure wrong, no incentives for consultants	1
Pay structure wrong, no incentives for GPs	*
Any mention of pay	**6**
Hours of work too long, too many nights and weekends	3
Any mention of pay or hours	**8**
Disappointed with career structure:	
Slow career progress	3
System of temporary registration (e.g. it impedes progress)	1
Standards vary — they are low at some hospitals	1
Status — would prefer to be independent of NHS with higher status	1
Any mention of career structure etc.	**6**

1 See note to Table IV. 6.

Looking at the sources of disappointment first in broad groupings, we find that 30 per cent of migrants are disappointed with job opportunities and 22 per cent with opportunities for study and training. Other sources of disappointment are comparatively unimportant, although 8 per cent of migrants mentioned pay or hours, and 6 per cent mentioned some aspect of the career structure or system.

Under the heading of job opportunities, one-fifth of migrants said simply that they could not get the job that they wanted, or that they could not get a good training job. A significant but small minority of migrants mentioned biassed selection or colour discrimination at this point in the interview, where the topic had not been raised by the interviewer. This shows that for the majority of migrants the general difficulty of finding a suitable job is more salient than biassed selection or colour discrimination, and that difficulties in finding a suitable job, though often mentioned, are not often spontaneously ascribed to bias or discrimination. Still under the heading of job opportunities, small proportions of migrants said that frequent job changes (which are the normal pattern for a junior doctor in the UK) were disruptive, that they had been forced to abandon their chosen specialty or field because they could not find an appropriate job, or that they were unable to get the particular sequence of jobs that would ideally make up the training programme for their specialty. These answers highlight the fact that a junior doctor's sequence of jobs is effectively a training programme, but one which he has to put together himself rather than one that is organised for him. Overseas doctors have difficulty, not merely in finding one suitable job, or in gaining access to one particular kind of training, but in putting together for themselves the appropriate programme of jobs and training combined.

Under the general heading of study and training, a small number of informants said that there was too little contact teaching or interplay of ideas with the consultant. Also, the examination system was criticised, not only because it fails many candidates, but also because there was said to be no guidance to those who had failed, or explanation of why they had failed, so that they were unable to concentrate on improving where they were particularly weak.

Job opportunities and opportunities for study and training were mentioned far more often than other sources of disappointment as Table IV. 9 shows. Eight per cent of migrants mentioned pay or hours of work (among whom 6 per cent mentioned pay). Only one per cent complained about the system of temporary registration.

The proportion of migrants who have found anything disappointing about studying or working in the UK is shown for a number of different sub-groups in Table A14. Looking at the analysis by country of qualification, we find that doctors from Arab countries are most likely to have complaints (69 per cent compared with 58 per cent for all adult migrants). Otherwise there is little difference between doctors from different areas. However, the actual complaints made vary widely between migrants who qualified in the UK or in a white anglophone country on the one hand, and overseas-qualified migrants apart from white anglophones on the other hand. (In racial terms, the former group is mostly white and the latter group mostly non-white.)

Complaints about job opportunities and opportunities for study and training are far more common among the majority of adult migrants who qualified outside the UK or a white anglophone country than among that minority who are British-qualified or from a white anglophone country. By contrast, those who are British-qualified or from a white

Table IV.10   Sources of disappointment with the UK (broad groupings) by country of qualification

		Percentages
	Country of qualification:		
	UK/Eire	White anglophone country	Elsewhere
Job opportunities	12	10	33
Study and training	12	7	24
Pay or hours	21	24	5
Others	9	10	6
Base: Adult migrants			
Unweighted	*61*	*66*	*889*
Weighted	*69*	*94*	*997*

anglophone country are far more likely than others to complain about pay or hours; this is a complaint that British doctors may well share, and which does not spring from the fact of being a migrant. The more important and characteristic complaints of overseas doctors are about job and training opportunities. Table IV.10 indicates that British-qualified and white anglophone doctors are less subject to these difficulties, probably because they are less racially and culturally distinct from the British, and because their qualifications, if not in fact British, are likely to be considered equivalent to British ones.

Among hospital doctors, those in geriatrics (72 per cent), general surgery (67 per cent) and gynaecology or obstetrics (67 per cent) are the most likely to have some disappointment to express. Although psychiatric specialties are generally thought to be unpopular and do contain a high concentration of overseas-qualified doctors, migrants in psychiatry are rather less likely than all migrants to have complaints (47 per cent of those in psychiatry have some disappointment to express).

The principal complaints of migrants in geriatrics are that they could not get the job they wanted or had to make many applications without success and that they could not get a good training job; 57 per cent of those in geriatrics mentioned one or other of these complaints, compared with only 19 per cent of those in specialties other than geriatrics, a ratio of three to one. This strongly suggests that the migrants who are now in geriatric jobs had, in many or most cases, hoped to do general medicine, but have taken jobs in geriatrics after failing to get the job in general medicine that they wanted. These informants rarely say that they have been forced to abandon the specialty of their choice because they still see geriatrics as broadly within the field of general medicine, although providing inadequate training and experience.

Very early migrants — those who came before 1960 — are rather less likely than the rest to have some disappointment to express. This confirms that these early migrants are a special group; many did not migrate for career reasons, and many obtained their primary qualifications in the UK. Recent migrants — those who came from 1973 on, and especially those who came in 1977 or 1978 — are also comparatively unlikely to have complaints, probably because they have yet to become disillusioned. However, we shall see that those who progress slowly and who fail to achieve their objectives are more likely to stay in this country. There should, therefore, be a relatively high proportion of successful doctors among the recent migrants, which could account for their tendency not to be disappointed.

It is also important to consider an analysis by language test score. If complaints are mostly made by doctors with inadequate English, then it can be argued that disappointments arise more from the doctors' own inadequacies than from the system which they are criticising. There is no support for this view from the proportion expressing any disappointment; in fact, migrants with better English are, if anything, more likely to have disappointments to express than those with poorer English. However, looking at the actual complaints made, we find that migrants with relatively low language test scores (up to 23) are rather more likely to complain about job opportunities than those with better scores (33 per cent compared with 22 per cent). Those with higher scores are more likely to complain about pay or hours instead. The difference is not very striking, but some of the migrants' difficulties do seem to be associated with imperfect English.

Among the aspects of studying and working in the UK that migrants found better than expected, several are the converse of the complaints that have just been considered. Thus 11 per cent mentioned high standards of training and teaching, a further 11 per cent good teaching facilities, libraries and access to laboratories, and a further 13 per cent praised other aspects of training and postgraduate education. It is notable, however, that no informants said that they had found it easier to get suitable jobs, or good training jobs, than they had expected, although as we have seen a substantial proportion mentioned difficulties in this field. A number of entirely fresh dimensions emerge on the positive side, which had not been mentioned on the negative side. For example, 6 per cent of migrants mentioned use and experience of advanced medicines, techniques or hardware, 6 per cent said their relationships with colleagues were better than they had expected and 5 per cent praised the discipline, organization, method or absence of confusion in the NHS, something which apparently contrasted with their expectations. (Table A14 shows the proportions finding something disappointing and better than expected among detailed sub-groups, and relates *passim* to the whole of the preceding section.)

Training and medical experience

The findings so far presented, which provide a general conspectus of how migrants compare their expectations with their experience, show that a substantial proportion have serious disappointments and criticisms to express, but also that a substantial proportion find that their experience has exceeded their expectations. Migrants' comments both on the positive and on the negative side tend to concentrate on training opportunities and on job opportunities seen as a principal determinant of training opportunities. To investigate this further, questions were included that concentrated on training specifically. From the answers to the broad question "Why did you come to Britain?" it is clear that the great majority of migrants came principally to gain postgraduate training and experience.

Table IV.11 What is better than expected about studying and working in the UK[1]

	Per cent
Training and teaching	
High standard of training and teaching/ higher than elsewhere	11
Teaching facilities, libraries, journals, access to laboratories	11
Many/well-designed courses	5
The content of training and teaching, e.g. more basic medical sciences, more on handling patients	4
Training and experience cover a wider range	2
Amount of contact teaching and supervision	2
More general answers on training, e.g. active educational programme	5
Job conditions	
Have time for study/leave for courses	7
Use and experience of advanced medicines, techniques or hardware	6
Good relationships with colleagues	6
Discipline/good organization/ no confusion/methodical system	5
Can study and work/learn and earn	3
People (doctors not specified) are friendly/helpful	1
Opportunities to do research	1
General answers praising the NHS or England	11
Other answers	3
Nothing better than expected	45

1 See note to Table IV. 6

A more specific question also establishes that the great majority (81 per cent) expected that opportunities for postgraduate medical training would be better in this country than in the country of origin.

In addition, migrants were asked whether they had obtained training in this country that they could not have obtained in the country of origin, and if so what kind of training. The questions were repeated for medical experience as opposed to training. Just over half of migrants said that they had obtained training and experience in the UK that they could not have obtained in the country of origin (training 59 per cent, experience 58 per cent). In relation to the findings that the great majority of migrants came to this country primarily to get medical training and experience, and that 81 per cent expected opportunities for postgraduate medical training to be better here than in the country of origin, these figures are low. They imply that at least one-fifth of migrants feel that they have not obtained the training or experience which they came especially to get, and which they expected to be available.

The unsatisfactory position of many overseas doctors in geriatrics is confirmed. Migrants in geriatrics are less likely to find that they have benefited from training that they could not have obtained at home than those in any other specialty. Those in anaesthetics and psychiatry are the most likely to take a positive view. In the case of psychiatry, this confirms the finding that, while the specialty may be thought of as unpopular, it is not one in which overseas doctors face unusual difficulties.

The results of these questions are not consistently related to the informants' language test scores (Table A15), which suggests that migrants' assessments of the training and experience that they have received in the UK are not a reflection of their capacity, by virtue of their language competence, to benefit from it.

When asked what kind of training they had received in this country that they could not have had in the country of origin, most informants answered in terms of a specialty or field, although there were also references to training in modern or advanced techniques (3 per cent), training in practical clinical, diagnostic or investigative medicine (4 per cent) and training in a broader range of procedures and techniques (3 per cent). The particular kinds of medical experience mentioned followed a similar pattern.

Most migrants (81 per cent) *expected* opportunities for postgraduate medical training to be better in this country than in the country of origin. When asked about the training opportunities actually available to them, 56 per cent said they were pleased with them, 33 per cent said they were disappointed, while the remaining 11 per cent had no definite opinion. This confirms the conclusion that a substantial minority of migrants have not had their expectations fulfilled with regard to the prime motive for the migration. Those who qualified in the UK or a white anglophone country are about half as likely to have been disappointed in their expectations in this respect as those who qualified elsewhere, which confirms

47

the view that difficulties in gaining access to postgraduate training are greatest for groups which are culturally and racially most distinct from British doctors, and whose basic qualifications are least likely to be considered equivalent to British ones.

Table IV.12 Whether pleased or disappointed by opportunities for postgraduate medical training in the UK (Q31)

Column percentages

	Total	Country of first qualification		
		UK/Eire	White anglophone country	Overseas (excluding white anglophones)
Pleased	56	54	72	54
Disappointed	33	23	17	35
Don't know/not relevant	11	23	11	11
Base: Adult migrants				
Unweighted	*1,016*	*61*	*66*	*889*
Weighted	*1,160*	*69*	*94*	*997*

Consistently with the earlier findings, migrants in geriatrics and general surgery tend to be most disappointed with training opportunities, while those in psychiatry tend to be most satisfied. There is again no consistent relationship with the language test score.

Career progress and salary

Migrants' expectations and experience as regards career progress and salary can also be compared, although these factors were not central to the decision to come to the UK in most cases. When directly asked whether their progress in medicine in the UK had been faster or slower than they expected, over one-third of migrants (36 per cent) said that their progress had been slower than expected, while 15 per cent said it had been faster than expected and 45 per cent the same as they expected. A fuller analysis is given in Table IV.13. Thus, a substantial proportion of migrants are disappointed with their progress, and those who are disappointed clearly outnumber those whose progress has exceeded their expectations. Those who qualified in the Indian sub-continent or an Arab country are four times as likely to be disappointed with their progress as those who qualified in a white anglophone country, and twice as likely as those who were born overseas but qualified in this country. This again demonstrates that cultural, racial and linguistic differences are more important than the mere fact of having qualified overseas.

Table IV.13   Career progress in the UK compared with expectations by country of first qualification

Column percentages

	Total	UK/ Eire	Country of first qualification:				
			White anglo- phone country	Indian sub- conti- nent	Arab country	Else- where	Overseas qualified (exclud- ing white anglo- phones)
Faster than expected	15	14	14	15	15	14	15
Slower than expected	36	22	11	41	44	27	39
As expected	45	52	70	41	40	49	42
Don't know	5	12	5	4	2	10	10
Base: Adult migrants							
Unweighted	*1,016*	*61*	*66*	*661*	*111*	*117*	*889*
Weighted	*1,160*	*69*	*94*	*741*	*119*	*137*	*997*

Q20 Has your progress in medicine in Britain been faster than you expected, slower than you expected, or about what you expected?

Those who came to the UK very recently and also those who came very early (up to 1959) are relatively unlikely to say that their progress has been slower than expected. The reason for this seems to be that it is too early yet for the recent migrants to assess their position, and the early migrants, are a special group, (many of whom migrated for political reasons and who therefore had different expectations) from different countries from the rest (for example, from continental Europe). Excluding early and late migrants, we find that among those who came to the UK between 1960 and 1976 39 per cent have progressed slower than expected, and the figure would rise still further if white anglophones and British-qualified migrants were excluded from this group. There is again no consistent relationship with language test score.

We have seen that rates of pay were an unimportant consideration in the decision to come to this country. Migrants did, however, tend to expect rates of pay for equivalent medical jobs to be higher here than in the country of origin, although there are large differences according to the country of origin of the migrants. White anglophones, in particular, very rarely either expected rates of pay to be higher in the UK or found that they were in fact higher. Doctors who were born abroad but qualified in the UK are also a special group in this context. It is more useful, therefore, to consider adult migrants apart from those who qualified in the UK or a white anglophone country. A substantial proportion (49 per

Table. IV.14 Salary expectations and experience (Qs 16-18)

Column percentages

	Expected rates of pay	Actual rates of pay of hospital doctors	Actual earnings of GPs
Pay or earnings:			
Higher in the UK	49	58	28
Higher in country of origin	10	13	28
About the same	17	18	13
No definite expectation/don't know	24	11	31
Base: Adult migrants excluding those who first qualified in the UK, Eire or a white anglophone country			
Unweighted	*889*	*889*	*889*
Weighted	*997*	*997*	*997*

cent) of these migrants expected rates of pay to be higher in the UK than in the country of origin—Table IV.14. A higher proportion found that rates of pay for hospital doctors were, in fact, higher (58 per cent), although a much lower proportion found that the rates of pay for general practitioners were higher (28 per cent). Doctors from the Indian sub-continent were particularly likely to expect and to find that rates of pay were higher in this country. Thus, overseas doctors think that they benefit from receiving rates of pay in the UK which are higher than they would have obtained at home for equivalent jobs, even though they have not generally come here for this reason.

Intended and actual length of stay
At the time when they came to the UK, the great majority of migrants intended to stay for a few weeks only. Of those who are still here, 30 per cent intended to stay for up to three years, 40 per cent for four to five years, 23 per cent for a longer or indeterminate period, and only 7 per cent permanently (Table IV.15). Of course, these figures do not indicate the intended length of stay of migrants arriving over a defined period, because many of those who intended to stay for a short period will have left the country, while those who intended to stay for longer will tend to have remained here. This means that the intended length of stay of all migrants arriving over a defined period would be still shorter.

If we consider the intended length of stay (again, of those who are still here) in relation to the actual length of stay to date, we find that most migrants have already stayed for substantially longer than they intended. Those who came to the UK up to 1959 have, to all intents and purposes,

Table IV.15   Intended length of stay on coming to the UK (Qs 33 and 34)

	Per cent
Up to 3 years	30
4 - 5 years	40
6 - 9 years	10
10 or more years	2
Did not intend to stay permanently, but don't know how long intended to stay	11
Permanently	7
Base: Adult migrants	
Unweighted	*1,016*
Weighted	*1,160*

remained permanently, but only 18 per cent of them originally intended to do so; the great majority (63 per cent) intended to stay for up to five years only. Those who came in 1960 to 1964 have stayed for at least 14 years, but 85 per cent of them intended to stay for five years or less. Those who came in 1965-69 have stayed for at least nine years, but 69 per cent of them intended to stay for five years or less. Thus, the great majority of migrants, whether from early or late years, originally intended to stay for a short period only, and most of those who are now in this country have either stayed for substantially longer than they meant to or have so far been here for only a short time.

Migrants who have stayed in the UK for longer than they originally intended give four principal reasons for doing so: (i) that they have not attained their educational, training or career objectives, or have progressed towards attaining them more slowly than they expected (37 per cent); (ii) that there are positive attractions about jobs, careers, or the style of medical practice in the UK (26 per cent); (iii) marriage or family circumstances (35 per cent); and (iv) political reasons that prevent them from retuning to the country of origin (16 per cent).

Thus a substantial proportion have stayed for longer than intended because of unexpected difficulties, and also a substantial proportion have stayed because of unexpected attractions of life in this country, but informants mentioning difficulties as a reason for staying outnumber those mentioning positive attractions (37 per cent compared with 26 per cent). One implication of this important finding is that the greater the difficulties of overseas doctors, and the more they tend to fail to achieve their educational and career objectives, the more likely they are to remain working within the NHS.

The importance of marriage or family circumstances as a reason for staying in the UK is not unexpected in the light of earlier findings. It was established that 27 per cent of adult migrants have married since first coming to this country, and that among all married adult migrants, 17

51

per cent of the men and 4 per cent of the women are married to a British person. These overseas doctors who have married a British person are probably strongly represented among those who have stayed for longer than they originally intended, of whom 35 per cent have stayed because they got married or for other family reasons.

Table IV.16   Reasons for staying in the UK for longer than originally intended, by type of job and language test score (Q37)

Percentages

	Total	Job type: GP	Hospital doctor	Overseas-qualified doctors by language test score: 0-18	19-25	26-29
Career and training difficulties:						
Did not pass exams, must get exams before returning	20	11	26	33	27	6
Could not get the training I wanted	17	8	23	27	13	10
I thought I would progress faster	3	1	5	1	5	1
Any career or training difficulties	37	19	49	56	42	17
Positive attractions of Britain:						
Attractions of jobs, career, life in Britain	23	24	22	15	20	33
Prefer the style of medical practice here	4	6	3	4	3	6
Any positive attraction	26	29	24	18	22	38
Other reasons:						
Got married/family reasons	35	50	24	26	30	46
Political reasons for not returning	16	15	17	19	11	14
Other reasons	6	9	3	3	6	5
Don't know	3	2	4	1	5	3
Base: Adult migrants who have stayed longer than intended						
Unweighted	*435*	*194*	*241*	*65*	*196*	*122*
Weighted	*486*	*208*	*278*	*73*	*211*	*138*

General practitioners are twice as likely as hospital doctors to have stayed for longer than intended because of marriage or family circumstances. It seems likely that in many cases the decision to remain in the UK because of marriage or family circumstances and the decision to switch to a career in general practice are one and the same decision, and this point will be discussed when the career path of GPs is considered in the next chapter. At the same time, GPs are comparatively unlikely to have stayed because of career or training difficulties (though 19 per cent have nevertheless done so).

Doctors with low language test scores (0-18) are more than three times as likely as those with high scores (26-29) to cite career or training difficulties as a reason for staying in this country for longer than intended. Those with high scores tend to have stayed because of the positive attractions or for family reasons. This is rather strong evidence that imperfect English is a factor preventing doctors from gaining the qualifications and training that would enable them to return home.

In the preceding discussion it has been assumed that migrants who did not originally intend to stay permanently in this country meant to return after a period to the country of origin. Although this is substantially true, 19 per cent of those who originally intended to leave after a period meant to go on to a different country rather than return home. The main countries which they intended to go to were the USA (four per cent), Canada (one per cent), Australia or New Zealand (two per cent) and countries in Asia (two per cent) or Africa (one per cent).

The qualifications and grade that migrants hoped to achieve

We have seen that the great majority of adult migrants (93 per cent) originally intended to leave the UK after a period. Of those who did not intend to stay permanently, the great majority (87 per cent) originally hoped to have one or more postgraduate medical qualifications before leaving. This applies to the great majority of those who are now GPs (80 per cent) as well as to those who are now hospital doctors (90 per cent). This is a further indication that most of those who have become GPs have done so after originally hoping to pursue a career in the hospital service.

This conclusion is strengthened when we consider the particular qualifications that migrants hoped to get. If percentages are based on those who did not originally intend to stay permanently, 65 per cent of GPs and 77 per cent of hospital doctors hoped to get membership or fellowship of a Royal College before leaving the UK (a qualification which the great majority of British GPs do not have or require); 20 per cent of GPs and 17 per cent of hospital doctors hoped to get a British postgraduate diploma.

Doctors from the Indian sub-continent or an Arab country are the most likely to have aspirations to membership or fellowship of a College (80 per cent and 86 per cent respectively); those from white anglophone countries are the least likely (49 per cent), nor did they often hope to get a diploma instead. This confirms the earlier conclusion that a significant proportion of white anglophones came to the UK as part of a 'grand tour' rather than primarily for medical training or experience. Migrants

C

who came at an earlier stage and qualified here are far more likely than other groups to have had a postgraduate degree as an objective (37 per cent). This small but significant group seems to consist of people from abroad who intended to pursue a career in teaching or research, and who came to this country for the whole of their medical training at undergraduate and postgraduate level.

Table IV.17   Qualifications that migrants hoped to get in the UK, by job type and country of first qualification

Percentages

	Type of job:		Country of first qualification:				
	GP	Hospital doctor	UK/ Eire	White anglo- phone country	Indian sub- con- tinent	Arab country	Else- where
Membership or Fellowship of a Royal College	65	77	37	49	80	86	66
Membership or Fellowship Part 1 only	1	2	7	1	1	2	1
Diploma	20	17	5	19	21	12	8
Postgraduate degree	3	4	37	2	2	3	3
Type not stated	6	3	5	2	4	5	3
None	20	10	32	31	7	6	26
Base: Adult migrants who did not intend to stay permanently							
Unweighted	*233*	*704*	*49*	*58*	*624*	*107*	*99*
Weighted	*251*	*822*	*57*	*86*	*700*	*111*	*119*

NB Fifteen per cent of all informants in this table mentioned *two* qualifications that they had hoped to get, hence columns add to over 100 per cent.

In short, migrants typically, although not universally, came to this country intending to pass the membership or fellowship examination within a few years, and then to retun to the country of origin. It is important to consider what proportion of those who had this typical plan have succeeded in their prime objective of getting the membership or fellowship qualification. table IV.18, which is based on those who had the typical plan, shows the proportion who have passed the membership or fellowship examination, and those who have passed Part 1 only, according to the year in which they came to the UK. Of those who came in 1969 or earlier (who have been here for at least nine years) less than half (46 per cent) have obtained membership or fellowship, while a further 8 per cent have passed the Part 1 examination only. Of those who came between 1970 and 1972 (who have been here for five to eight years) 35 per cent have membership or fellowship, and a further 15 per cent have Part 1 only. Those who came in more recent years have not yet had very long to gain the necessary experience and study for the examinations; it is not therefore surprising to find that a relatively small proportion have yet passed them.

Table IV.18 Proportion of adult migrants with Membership or Fellowship of a Royal College, by year of migration

Per cent

	Up to 1959	1960-1969	Up to 1969[1]	1970-1972	Up to 1972[1]	1973-1974	1975-1978
			Year of coming to the UK:				
Membership/Fellowship	37	50	46	35	43	23	8
Membership/Fellowship —Part 1 only	8	7	8	15	10	20	18
Base: Adult migrants *Weighted*	*65*	*214*	*279*	*110*	*389*	*170*	*214*

1 These columns are subtotals of previous columns.

Because those who successfully achieve their objectives are probably more likely to leave the country, these figures are difficult to interpret. They show that of doctors who had the typical plan and who are still in this country, less than half have achieved the prime objective of obtaining membership or fellowship, even if we consider only those who have had nine years or more in which to do so. It is a fact, therefore, that upwards of half of migrants who have been here for nine years or more have failed in their own terms. But this is not to say that half of those who come over a defined period are destined to fail, because the successful ones are probably more likely to leave within a short period. Unfortunately, there is no reliable method of converting the information that we have about the stock of doctors into information about the flow.

Adult migrants who did not originally intend to stay permanently in the UK generally hoped to reach registrar (46 per cent) or senior registrar level (21 per cent) before leaving; they rarely hoped to reach consultant level (7 per cent). The remaining 27 per cent either had no definite expectations as to grade, or (rarely) intended to work as GPs before leaving.

If we consider those who expected to reach registrar level before leaving the UK (Tables A19 and A20), we find that, among those who came nine or more years ago, only 5 per cent are at a level below registrar, 16 per cent are registrars, and 27 per cent are at a level above registrar. However, 49 per cent have, in fact become GPs instead of leaving this country on reaching registrar level. Thus, a substantial proportion have changed their original intention, either by staying on as GPs, or by progressing in the hospital service to a higher level than they had intended tc before leaving. The same is true of those who intended to leave after reaching senior registrar level or above.

We shall be able to understand these comparisons between intentions and experience more fully when we have considered career progress in a general way in the next chapter.

V Career Progress

Overseas-qualified doctors, as has already been mentioned, are strongly concentrated in the lower grades of the hospital service and they tend to be working in specialties that are generally considered to be unpopular. Although the great majority came to the UK to obtain medical training and experience which they could not easily get in their country of origin, there is a strong tendency for them to be working in 'non-teaching' health districts rather than in the teaching districts where training opportunities are likely to be superior. Many are dissatisfied with their training opportunities and career progress, and have failed to achieve their own objectives within the expected timetable. Of those who have been in the UK for more than a few years, most have stayed longer than they intended, often because they have not yet achieved their objectives. These findings may seem to suggest that overseas-qualified doctors face special difficulties, which are not shared by British-qualified doctors, in gaining access to suitable medical experience and training, in acquiring postgraduate medical qualifications, and in progressing to higher levels in the career structure.

However, we have so far taken only a very partial view of the matter. We have considered the aims, objectives and disappointments of migrants, but British doctors may also fail to achieve their objectives and may also be disappointed as a result. Also, the age structure of overseas-qualified doctors as a group is radically different from that of British-qualified doctors. Overseas-qualified doctors (particularly those in the hospital service) are mainly concentrated in the 30-44 age group, so that comparatively few have reached the age at which they might be expected to occupy the more senior posts. As might also be expected from this age profile, a comparatively small proportion of overseas-qualified doctors possess postgraduate medical qualifications, particularly membership or fellowship of a Royal College. Although this could partly be a consequence of a lack of training opportunity, it could also partly account for the concentration of overseas doctors in the lower grades. While a majority of overseas-qualified doctors have a good command of English, an important minority do not, and this could account for a failure to gain access to suitable training and experience or to benefit from it, and consequently to make good career progress.

In this chapter we shall attempt a more rigorous analysis of the career progress of British and overseas-qualified doctors in order to assess how far overseas-qualified doctors face special difficulties and what these difficulties are. We shall start by comparing the original career preferences and specialty choices of the two groups and the extent to which they have achieved their original objectives. Secondly, we shall compare the actual career histories of the two groups. Finally, we shall analyse the present position of overseas and British-qualified doctors, making allowances for the large differences between the two groups in terms of age, command of English and level of qualification.

Choice of career

Whether they are to become hospital doctors or general practitioners all doctors share the same kind of undergraduate medical training, and after taking the Bachelor of Medicine (MB) examinations, spend one year working at house officer level in the hospital service before they become eligible for full registration. At this point the GP and hospital careers begin to diverge. In the past there was no statutory requirement that GPs should have undergone special training, although those who had two years' specified postgraduate hospital experience and one year's training in general practice became eligible for a special training allowance which increased their total remuneration. Regulations now being phased in will eventually require (probably by 1982) that GP principals should have undergone a three-year training programme of general practice and hospital training (already a majority of doctors now entering general practice have undergone a training programme of this kind). However, in the recent past, what happened was that some members of a cohort of junior doctors would simply peel off each year and go into general practice. Some of a given cohort would thus become GPs at the first opportunity (one, or more often, two years after graduation) while others would move to general practice at a later stage after having gained further experience in the hospital service, and maybe having given up an earlier intention to pursue a specialist career.

Those who are hoping to pursue a career within the hospital service will normally decide on a specialty after the pre-registration year (if not before) and will then try to work in a series of junior jobs which together will give them the appropriate range of training and experience. An important objective will be to pass the membership or fellowship examination for the chosen specialty, and the junior doctor's series of jobs must at least meet the requirements set by the relevant Royal College for eligibility to sit the examination. An appropriate range of jobs will include experience of related specialties as well as all relevant aspects of the chosen one.

General practice and the hospital service can therefore be seen as two related but widely divergent careers starting from a common point. After the decision to study medicine, the most important decision that a doctor takes is whether to become a GP or aim to become a consultant.

In order to investigate the choice between the two main medical careers, all informants in the survey were asked 'At the time when you passed the MB did you hope to become a specialist or a GP, or did you plan some other career?'. The findings show that only 17 per cent of doctors had no definite preference at this stage; just over half (53 per cent) hoped to become specialists and 28 per cent expected to become GPs. Analysis by the actual career suggests that specialist careers are more sought after than careers in general practice, since 31 per cent of GPs originally hoped to be specialists, whereas only 11 per cent of hospital doctors hoped to be GPs (and most of this latter group are junior hospital doctors who will in fact become GPs within a year or two). Thus, there is substantial switching from the hospital service to general practice, but very little movement in the opposite direction.

We have shown in earlier chapters that the great majority of overseas-qualified doctors came to the UK for postgraduate medical training that is available in the hospital service and that is fundamentally a preparation for a career as a specialist rather than as a GP. It is not, therefore, surprising to find that the great majority of overseas-qualified doctors (89 per cent excluding white anglophones) originally hoped to become specialists, compared with a much smaller proportion of the British-qualified (42 per cent). British-qualified doctors comprise a broad spec-

Table V.1 Preferred career at the time of passing the MB, by present post and country of qualification.

Column percentages

	Total	Present post:		Country of qualification:		
		GPs	Hospital Doctors	UK/Eire	White anglo-phones	Elsewhere
Specialist	53	31	69	42	48	89
General practitioners	28	50	11	33	31	8
Other career	3	3	2	3	6	1
No definite preference	17	16	21	21	15	2
Base: All informants						
Unweighted	*1,981*	*730*	*1,251*	*1,016*	*73*	*892*
Weighted	*4,490*	*1,923*	*2,567*	*3,382*	*104*	*1,004*

Q 61 At the time when you passed your MB did you hope to become a specialist or a GP, or did you plan some other career?

trum, whereas overseas-qualified doctors are a self-selected group including only those who hoped to pursue a career at a high level as a specialist and who were prepared to go abroad to gain the necessary training. Doctors from white anglophone countries are like British-qualified doctors in this respect: a substantial proportion of them (31 per cent) originally intended to become GPs.

Medical services and consequently career structures may be different in the countries of origin, where private practice generally has far more importance than in the UK, and where a doctor in private practice may combine some of the functions of specialist and GP. The overseas-qualified doctors' answers to the survey question show that most of them intended to specialise, although the context in which they would work as specialists might be very different from what it is in this country.

Table V.2 Preferred career at the time of passing the MB by country of qualification: GPs and hospital doctors

Column percentages

	Total	GPs qualified in:			Hospital doctors qualified in:		
		UK/ Eire	White anglo- phone country[1]	Else- where	UK/ Eire	White anglo- phone country	Else- where
Specialist	53	24	(2)	78	60	57	92
General prac- titioners	28	54	(14)	18	13	23	5
Other career	3	4	(1)	1	3	6	1
No definite preference	17	18	(3)	3	25	14	1
Base: All informants							
Unweighted	*1,981*	*477*	*13*	*240*	*539*	*60*	*652*
Weighted	*4,490*	*1,649*	*20*	*255*	*1,733*	*84*	*749*

1 In this column, the figures are numbers and not percentages

Q61 At the time when you passed your MB did you hope to become a specialist or a GP, or did you plan some other career?

General practitioners may be divided into those who originally intended to become GPs, and those who originally intended to become specialists and switched to general practice later. Among British-qualified GPs, those who made a later decision to pursue this career account for 24 per cent of the total, whereas among overseas-qualified GPs (excluding white anglophones), they are the great majority (78 per cent). This confirms indications in earlier chapters that overseas-qualified doctors who become GPs tend to do so reluctantly after first trying to pursue a career in the hospital service. As most overseas-qualified doctors, when they come to the UK, intend to return to their country of origin within a few years, those who become GPs may have made a simultaneous decision to remain here and to work in general practice instead of returning to the country of origin to work as a specialist. It was shown in the last chapter that 50 per cent of overseas-qualified GPs decided to remain in the UK for family reasons; these doctors may have first and foremost made the decision to remain (for example, because they had married a British person), but may then have decided that their best career within the British context would be in general practice, whereas they would have become specialists if they had returned to the country of origin. However, this kind of explanation can only apply, at a maximum, to half of the overseas-qualified GPs. For the remainder, a failure to progress as expected within the hospital service may have been the main reason for entering general practice against the original intention.

Choice of specialty

After the choice of general practice or the hospital service, the next important decision, for those preferring a career in the hospital service, is the choice of specialty. We have seen in an earlier chapter that the actual

Table V.3   **Preferred specialty compared with actual distribution of hospital posts by specialty (Q62)**

		Percentages
	Preferred[1]	Actual[2]
Paediatrics	7	5
Geriatrics	0.5	5
General medicine	21	12
Other medical specialties	5	6
All medical specialties less geriatrics	33	22
General surgery	25	10
Other surgical specialties	6	13
All surgical specialties	30	23
Anaesthetics	5	11
Radiology/radiotherapy	2	6
Gynaecology/obstetrics	12	8
Pathology specialties	5	7
Psychiatry specialties	5	9
Accident and emergency	0.5	3
Other specialties	7	5

1 Some informants mentioned more than one preferred specialty and some had no definite preference. Percentages are based on all *mentions* of a particular specialty. Base: 2,373 (weighted)
2 The actual distribution (from the survey for comparability) is based on hospital doctors whose specialty is known (for 3% the information is not available). Base: 2,474 (weighted) or approximately 1,250 (unweighted)

distribution of overseas doctors across specialties is different from that of British doctors, and it was suggested that the overseas doctors tended to be concentrated in the less popular specialties, although there was no definite indication at that stage as to which specialties were comparatively unpopular. We can now examine this question in greater depth by comparing the preferred specialty at the time of passing the MB with the actual distribution across specialties. Doctors who at the time of passing the MB hoped to become specialists were asked what specialty they had hoped to pursue. Popular specialties can be defined as those for which the proportion of doctors who originally hoped to work in them is higher than the proportion who actually work in them, and unpopular specialties conversely. Table V.3 shows that the most popular specialties in this sense are general medicine, general surgery and gynaecology/obstetrics. The least popular specialties are geriatrics, anaesthetics, radiology/radiotherapy and psychiatry. Surgical specialties other than general surgery also appear to be relatively unpopular, although this may be misleading, in that a doctor who hopes to practice as a surgeon may think at an early stage in terms of general surgery simply because he makes little distinction between the various surgical specialties. If we group all surgical specialties together we find that they are popular as a group (more doctors prefer them than work in them).

The findings just quoted are a direct measure of the popularity of the various specialties among doctors included in the survey. The Department of Health and Social Security (DHSS) regularly reviews career prospects in the various specialties, which it considers to be mostly dependent on their relative popularity, although other factors also have an influence (for example, the rate of growth of specialties and the age distribution of doctors already in them). In order to assess career prospects, the DHSS compiles statistics of the number of applications and candidates per post, for consultant and senior registrar posts in the various specialties. Roughly speaking, specialties having a higher than average number of applicants per post ought to be the popular ones, and those with a lower than average number ought to be the unpopular ones. The survey findings on popularity are in close agreement with the DHSS statistics on fields of recruitment, although figures are not available from the survey for the smallest specialties.[1]

Taking this analysis a step further, we can consider the preferred and actual distribution across specialties for British and overseas-qualified doctors separately. The original specialty preferences of the two groups are broadly similar as shown in Table V.4. However, overseas-qualified doctors are more likely than British-qualified doctors to have preferred a surgical specialty or gynaecology/obstetrics, and less likely to have preferred a pathology specialty. These differences in preferences between

---

1 For DHSS statistics for a period comparable with the survey, see Health Trends, August 1978, No. 3, Vol 10, page 61.

the two groups are unrelated to the differences in the actual distribution across specialties. It is clear, therefore, that overseas-qualified doctors are concentrated in certain specialties not because they originally preferred those specialties but for some other reason. In fact, the gap between original preferences and actual specialisation is greater for overseas-qualified than for British-qualified doctors.

Table V.4 Preferred specialty compared with actual distribution of hospital posts, by specialty, for British and overseas-qualified doctors separately (Q62)

Column percentages

	Qualified UK/Eire		Qualified elsewhere	
	Preferred[1]	Actual[2]	Preferred[1]	Actual[2]
Paediatrics	7	5	7	3
Geriatrics	1	2	*	10
General medicine	23	14	18	7
Other medical specialties	4	6	6	4
All medical specialties less geriatrics	34	26	31	15
General surgery	22	11	28	9
Other surgical specialties	4	10	8	17
All surgical specialties	26	21	36	27
Anaesthetics	4	10	6	13
Radiology/radiotherapy	3	8	2	4
Gynaecology/obstetrics	10	8	15	10
Pathology specialties	8	8	2	4
Psychiatry specialties	5	8	4	10
Accident and emergency	1	3	*	4
Other specialties	8	6	4	5

1 Some informants mentioned more than one preferred specialty and some had no definite preference. Percentages are based on all *mentions* of a particular specialty. Weighted bases are 1,414 (British-qualified) and 959 (overseas-qualified)
2 The actual distribution is based on British-qualified or overseas-qualified hospital doctors whose specialty is known. Bases are: British-qualified, 1,670 (weighted) and 530 approx. (unweighted); overseas-qualified, 801 (weighted) and 710 approx. (unweighted).

It can be seen that the ratio between the percentage of doctors preferring each of these specialties and the percentage actually working in them is higher among overseas-qualified than among British-qualified doctors. The converse is true of geriatrics. Less than 0.5 per cent of overseas-qualified doctors originally hoped to specialise in geriatrics, whereas ten per cent of them are working in that specialty; one per cent of British-qualified doctors originally preferred geriatrics, and two per cent are working in it.

This analysis shows that the balance of supply and demand varies considerably between specialties so that doctors, whatever their country of qualification, often have to modify their choice of specialty in the light of the opportunities available. While the initial specialty preferences of overseas doctors are broadly similar to those of British doctors, overseas doctors are more likely to have to settle for a second-choice specialty, and therefore tend to be concentrated in the specialties that are, generally speaking, less popular.

Progress towards objectives
In the last chapter we considered how overseas doctors evaluate their actual progress in relation to their expectations on coming to the UK, and we found that a substantial proportion of those who have not returned to the country of origin and who are therefore in the UK at a given time had failed to achieve their objectives within the timetable they had set themselves. However, it was not clear how far these disappointments might be shared with British doctors.

In order to make possible direct comparisons between British and overseas doctors, all informants were also asked whether, in terms of further study and examinations, they had progressed as fast as they originally expected to, and if not, what had caused their progress to be slower than expected. Twenty per cent of British-qualified doctors, 27 per cent of white anglophones and 55 per cent of other overseas-qualified doctors said they had progressed slower than they expected. This shows that overseas doctors are substantially more likely than British ones to perceive their progress towards study objectives as slow, and confirms that the special disappointments encountered by overseas doctors from most countries are shared to only a limited extent by those from white anglophone countries. While there is a strong contrast between white anglophone and other overseas doctors, differences between those from the Indian sub-continent, Arab countries and elsewhere are slight.

Among the reasons given for having progressed more slowly than expected the most important are lack of time for study (17 per cent of overseas-qualified doctors excluding white anglophones), failure in examinations (7 per cent) and inability to get a good training job or an otherwise suitable job (15 per cent), but a wide range of other reasons are also given. Discrimination or lack of equal opportunity is mentioned by two per cent of overseas-qualified doctors (excluding anglophones) and not at all by white anglophones (Table A21).

Overseas-qualified hospital doctors and GPs are equally likely to feel that they have progressed more slowly than they expected. A particularly high proportion of overseas-qualified doctors with no postgraduate qualification (65 per cent) have been disappointed in their expectations, compared with 34 per cent of those with membership or fellowship of a Royal college. At the same time, this shows that one-third of those who now have membership or fellowship nevertheless feel that they progressed to that point more slowly than expected. This compares with 12 per cent of British-qualified doctors with membership or fellowship.

Table V.5   Proportion who have progressed slower than expected in terms of further study and examinations (Q68)

Percentages

	Qualified in UK/Eire	All overseas-qualified
Highest qualification		
Membership or Fellowship	12	34
Membership or Fellowship -		
Part 1 only	20	56
British Diploma	21	53
Other qualification	20	42
No postgraduate qualification	27	65
Language test score		
0-18	n.a.	57
19-23	20	59
24-29	20	37

NB The base for each cell in the table is different; neither columns nor rows are therefore additive.

From the reasons given for staying for longer than originally intended (see Chapter IV) it seems likely that overseas doctors who achieve their training objectives within a reasonable period of time tend to return quickly to the country of origin, and that the extent of dissatisfaction is, therefore, exaggerated by a tendency for the unsuccessful to remain and form part of the population sampled. Some of the force is taken from this argument by an analysis of postgraduate qualifications. The gap between the British and overseas-qualified in satisfaction with speed of progress is just as great among those who have passed the membership or fellowship examinations as among those at lower levels of qualification. It is not just a group of overseas doctors who have failed to achieve their objectives who are dissatisfied with their progress; those who have achieved their objectives are also dissatisfied. It is still true that those who achieved their objectives *quickly* may be under-represented in a sample of the stock.

Analysis by command of English shows that overseas doctors with very high test scores (24 or more) are substantially less likely to be dissatisfied with their progress than those with lower scores, and at first sight this seems to imply that inadequate English is a major cause of slow progress. Against this, a number of points can be made. First, there is no difference between those with low scores (0-18) and those with middling to good ones (19-23), whereas we would expect those with definitely poor English to have progressed particularly slowly. Secondly, the evidence given in the chapter on command of English suggests that those with scores between 19 and 23 tend to have little linguistic disadvantage, yet they are substantially more dissatisfied with their progress than those with higher scores. Thirdly, and most important, a significant number of British-qualified doctors scored between 19 and 23 on the test, and they appear to be no more dissatisfied with their progress than British-qualified doctors scoring 24-29, whereas in the case of overseas-qualified doctors there is a decisive difference between these two groups.

Thus, in the case of overseas-qualified doctors there is a clear relationship between command of English and satisfaction with career progress which, however, does not apply to British-qualified doctors at all. In addition, we find that overseas-qualified doctors with low language test scores are more likely than those with high scores to give inability to get good training jobs and lack of time for study as reasons for slow progress, whereas again the same is not true of British-qualified doctors. A possible explanation of these findings is that where doctors are overseas-qualified, minor features of their spoken English will tend to assume significance for selection committees and to be used as a criterion for selection, but where doctors are British-qualified small linguistic differences will not be noticed.

The great majority of hospital doctors (89 per cent) expected to obtain some postgraduate qualification within ten years of passing the MB examinations, and nearly two-thirds (63 per cent) expected to obtain membership or fellowship of a Royal College within this period. A rather higher proportion of overseas-qualified hospital doctors (71 per cent) than of British-qualified (60 per cent) expected to obtain membership or fellowship within ten years. This provides further confirmation of the finding that overseas-qualified doctors tend to be highly motivated towards further study. A much higher proportion of overseas-qualified GPs (60 per cent) than of British-qualified GPs (30 per cent) expected to obtain membership or fellowship within ten years of passing the MB.

Table V.6   Doctors with Membership or Fellowship as proportion of those who expected to obtain Membership or Fellowship within ten years of qualifying (Qs 66 and 67)

Percentages

	Doctors who qualified up to 10 years ago:		Doctors who qualified more than 10 years ago:	
	British-qualified	Overseas-qualified	British-qualified	Overseas-qualified
With Membership/ Fellowship	32	16	52	38
With Membership/ Fellowship - Part 1 only	14	19	4	9
Weighted base	*632*	*367*	*888*	*349*

This fits in with the finding that a high proportion of overseas-qualified GPs had originally intended to pursue a career as a specialist.

Considering only those (whether now GPs or hospital doctors) who expected to obtain membership or fellowship within ten years of graduation, we can now compare the proportions of the British and overseas-qualified who have achieved that objective. In making this comparison, it is also useful to look separately at those who graduated within the past ten years and those who graduated more than ten years ago. The latter group should by now have obtained membership or fellowship if they have achieved their original objective to the expected timetable. In fact, 52 per cent of the British-qualified and 38 per cent of the overseas-qualified have done so. This shows that there is a significant, though not very substantial, tendency for overseas doctors to fail to achieve their study objective more often than British ones. Among those who graduated less than ten years ago and expected to obtain membership or fellowship within ten years, 32 per cent of the British-qualified and 16 per cent of the overseas-qualified have already passed the membership or fellowship examinations. This sharper difference suggests that overseas doctors are substantially less likely than British ones to obtain membership or fellowship within a relatively short period from graduation, or that those who pass it quickly tend to return rapidly to the country of origin.

Table V.7 Grade of the last job abroad compared with the first job in the UK

		Column percentages
	Last job abroad	First job in the UK
General practitioners	13	2
Hospital doctors		
House officer	17	16
Senior house officer	18	63
Registrar	31	9
Senior registrar	3	*
Medical assistant	1	*
Consultant	1	*
Grade not stated	8	9
Other type of job	1	—
No information	8	*
Base: Overseas doctors who previously practised abroad		
Unweighted	*855*	*855*
Weighted	*979*	*979*

Effect of migration on career history

There was a marked tendency for those migrants who had already practised abroad to lose seniority on coming to the UK. Only 12 per cent of
overseas-qualified doctors migrated to the UK immediately after passing
the MB or equivalent. Among those who had already practised abroad,
we find that 36 per cent last worked as registrars (or above) abroad; only
9 per cent started at registrar level or above in the UK and whereas only
18 per cent last worked at senior house officer level abroad, 63 per cent
started at this level in the UK.

The immediate effect of the migration on doctors' seniority can be
more closely examined through cross-analysis of the grade of the last job
abroad and the first job in this country as shown in Table V.8. Of those
who last worked as GPs abroad, the great majority went into the hospital
service in this country, mostly at senior house officer (63 per cent) or
house officer level (18 per cent). It is difficult to make comparisons in
terms of seniority between GPs and hospital doctors, but it seems fair to
say that the 18 per cent of former GPs who started in the UK as house officers had slipped back to some extent. Those who last worked as
registrars abroad, were the largest single group, accounting for 31 per
cent of migrants, but only 13 per cent started at the same grade in the
UK, while 68 per cent slipped back to senior house officer and 10 per cent
slipped back to house officer.

Table V.8   Grade of the first job in the UK by grade of the last job abroad

Column percentages

	\ Grade of last job abroad:				
	GP	HO	SHO	Registrar	SR/MA/ Consult- ant
Grade of first job in the UK					
General practitioner	5	1	1	1	—
House officer	18	27	16	10	10
Senior house officer	63	62	74	68	43
Registrar	5	2	4	13	31
Senior registrar/Medical assistant/Consultant	2	—	—	*	7
Not stated	8	7	6	7	10
Base: Overseas qualified doctors who previous practised abroad *Weighted*		164	179	304	42

NB Informants for whom the grade of the last job abroad is not known are excluded from
this table.

One way of summarising these findings is to say that migrants tend to start in the UK as senior house officers regardless of the grade they had previously reached abroad. This means that those who had previously held junior posts do best, either moving forward to the next grade or maintaining their position, while those who had previously held senior posts do worst and typically slip back one or more grades. This implies that selection committees pay little regard to an applicant's experience abroad. It seems that an overseas doctor on arrival can expect to get a house officer or senior house officer post regardless of his previous experience, but is unlikely to get any post at a higher grade.

An alternative analysis, in terms of time periods, demonstrates this rather more simply. Overseas-qualified doctors who start at senior house officer level in the UK have, on average, worked previously for 53 months abroad, whereas British-qualified doctors work, on average, for 22 months before reaching senior house officer level. The equivalent figures for registrar level are 78 months for overseas-qualified doctors and 46 months for British-qualified doctors. Both groups of overseas doctors lose almost exactly the same amount of time compared with British doctors — 31 months in the case of those starting as senior house officers, and 32 months in the case of those starting as registrars.

These findings show that one important immediate effect of the migration is that overseas doctors lose seniority and time. For those who eventually achieve their objectives in coming to this country, this may be a price worth paying, but for those who do not it must underline their failure. It could be argued that, because of the lack of equivalence between career structures in different countries, and because of the problems of adaptation shared by all migrants, some backwards movement at the time of the migration is inevitable. Also, it may be said that overseas doctors are best suited for the grades of post in which they start in the UK in spite of their apparently greater seniority in the country of origin. We were not able to investigate these questions further. However, what we shall later consider is whether the current position of overseas-qualified doctors, a position that is partly determined by the slippage at the time of the migration, is justified by the totality of their experience, qualifications and linguistic competence.

Time spent in reaching the present grade

We know that overseas-qualified doctors tend to lose time when they migrate, but they could, in principle, catch up again later to overcome their initial disadvantages on coming to the UK, or alternatively they could fall further behind. We can investigate this question by considering the total time spent from passing the MB examinations to the date of interview and relating this to the doctor's present grade. We find that overseas-qualified doctors who are now at senior house officer level have, on average, worked for 93 months since passing the MB examinations, whereas British-qualified senior house officers have worked for an average of 30 months. In the case of registrars and senior registrars, the gap between the two groups is smaller, though still substantial. It is interesting to note that the total time worked by British-qualified registrars is actually ten months shorter than that worked by overseas-qualified senior house officers. These findings show that overseas doctors do not generally later retrieve the time that they lose at the time of the migration. Those who have progressed to registrar or senior registrar are still more than 30 months behind their British-qualified counterparts, while those who are still at SHO level show a definite tendency to fall further behind. It seems that there is a sub-group of overseas doctors who, having started in the UK, usually at senior house officer level, have great difficulty in progressing to a higher grade.

Table V.9   Months since passing the MB by present grade:
British and overseas-qualified hospital doctors compared

	British-qualified	Overseas-qualified
Present grade:		
House officer	13	n.a.
Senior house officer	30	93
Registrar	83	118
Senior registrar	128[1]	167[1]

1 Low base

Notes:
1 The figures shown are average (mean) months.
2 The period defined is from passing the MB examinations to the month of interview, and in the case of the overseas doctors includes time spent abroad before coming to the UK.
3 The base for each mean is different, and is all British or overseas-qualified doctors now at the relevant hospital grade.
4 Figures are not given for consultants, because they would not be comparable (since consultants cannot be promoted further). Figures are not given for medical assistants, because bases are too low.

The fact that the law did not provide for full registration to be granted to temporarily registered doctors could be taken to imply that their qualifications or experience are in some way considered to be inferior. From this, it could be argued that the relatively slow progress of overseas-qualified doctors was, in fact, confined to those who had at first (or were still) temporarily registered, and that slow progress among this group was understandable and justifiable. However, further analysis shows that, if anything, the opposite is the case. Overseas-qualified doctors whose first registration in the UK was temporary, have on average reached their present grade more quickly than those whose first registration was full or provisional.

Table V.10 Months since passing the MB by present grade: overseas-qualified doctors by first type of registration

| | First registration in Britain: | |
	Temporary	Full or provisional
Present grade:		
Senior house officer	90	98
Registrar	108	126

Notes:
1 See notes 1 and 2 on Table V.10
2 The base for each mean is all overseas-qualified doctors at the stated grade and with the stated registration history.
3 Figures are not given for consultant because they would not be comparable, and not for the other grades because bases are too low.

Time spent between various stages of the career in the UK

We know that overseas doctors lose time when they migrate and also that they subsequently tend to fall further behind rather than to catch up. We can also establish how long they take to climb the various steps of the career ladder in this country. For example, we can define a group of doctors who have been house officers and who are now at registrar level or above, and for this group we can establish the average length of time taken to progress from house officer to registrar. A similar analysis can be done for any pair of grades (provided that the relevant doctors are a large enough group for separate analysis). What has to be remembered when considering the results of this kind of analysis is that only doctors who have, in fact, progressed are being considered. There may be a further group of doctors who have remained in their initial grade, and we shall consider this group shortly.

The findings show that among overseas-qualified doctors who do progress, the rate of progress is fairly similar to that of British doctors, although one relatively numerous group, those who start in this country as SHOs, do progress relatively rather more slowly. These differences in rate of progress once established in this country are far less important than the time lost between the last job abroad and the first job in the UK.

But we should not forget that there is a group of overseas doctors who have not progressed at all since coming here. The importance of this group can be seen from an analysis of months worked in the present grade. British-qualified senior house officers have, on average, been senior house officers for 16 months, whereas for overseas-qualified

Table V.11   Months between various points of the career in the UK: Overseas and British-qualified doctors compared

	British-qualified	Overseas-qualified
House officer to Senior house officer	22	15
House officer to Registrar	46	39
House officer to Senior registrar	89	78[1]
House officer to Consultant	139	122[2]
Senior house officer to Registrar	25	32
Senior house officer to Senior registrar	64	70
Senior house officer to Consultant	106	126[1]
Registrar to Senior registrar	46	46
Registrar to Consultant	90	85

1 Low base (under 50)
2 Low base (under 30)

Notes:
1 The figures given are average (mean) periods in months.
2 The periods run from the beginning of the first job in the first grade to the beginning of the first job in the second.
3 The date of starting in the first grade in the UK is counted as the starting point; overseas doctors may of course have already worked in an equivalent or higher grade abroad.
4 For each defined period only doctors who have worked at both of the relevant grades in the hospital service in the UK are counted.

senior house officers[2] the comparable figure is 31 months (counting time in the UK only) or almost twice as long. In the case of registrars, the difference while still significant, is much less marked: British-qualified registrars have worked as registrars for 28 months on average, compared with 34 months for overseas-qualified registrars.[3]

In this last analysis, all doctors at senior house officer or registrar level are included, whether or not they have progressed from a previous grade. When we look at the matter in this light, we do find that there is a tendency, strong in the case of senior house officers, for overseas doctors to have worked longer in their present grade than British ones. At the same time, there is comparatively little tendency for the rate of progress of those overseas doctors who have progressed to be slower than that of British doctors who have progressed through the same stages. It follows that there is a group of overseas doctors who get stuck, particularly at senior house officer level, and it is mainly (though not entirely) in this

2 The figures for SHOs are based on those who are now SHOs and whose first SHO post was in the UK, and similarly for registrars. Thus the period referred to is that spent in the present grade in the UK since reaching this grade.
3 Forty-two per cent of overseas qualified doctors are SHOs and 31 per cent are registrars. These figures represent, therefore, the experience of a majority of overseas qualified doctors.

sense that overseas doctors as a group tend to fall further behind after having already lost time between the last job abroad and the first one in the UK.

Career path of GPs

A great deal of evidence has already accumulated to show that overseas doctors who become GPs in this country tend to do so reluctantly, after having first tried to pursue a career in the hospital service. First, the great majority of overseas doctors come to the UK to obtain postgraduate qualifications which are mainly useful for a specialist career. Secondly, a much higher proportion of overseas-qualified than of British-qualified GPs have passed the membership or fellowship examinations. Thirdly, most overseas-qualified GPs say that they originally meant to be specialists, whereas the same is not true of the majority of British-qualified GPs. At the same time, it may be that many overseas-qualified GPs decided to settle permanently in the UK for reasons unconnected with their careers, and then decided that general practice was a more appropriate career for them within the British context.

Table V.12   Time spent working as a hospital doctor before becoming a GP

Percentages

	British-qualified	Overseas-qualified	
		Time spent abroad or in the UK	Time spent in the UK
None	—	—	6
18 months	23	2	11
19-36 months	26	3	15
Over 3 to 6 years	30	21	30
Over 6 to 10 years	12	32	20
Over 10 years	4	33	8
Not stated	6	8	10
Mean months	44	99	60
Base: All GPs			
Unweighted	*472*	*246*	
Weighted	*1,641*	*264*	

We can provide more specific information on this issue by considering the point at which GPs left the hospital service for general practice. Among British-qualified GPs, 59 per cent entered general practice after up to three years in the hospital service; these can be regarded as mainstream entrants to general practice. The group of somewhat late entrants, who went into general practice after three to six years, accounts for 30 per cent, while 12 per cent went into general practice after six to ten years, and 4 per cent after more than ten years. In broad terms, therefore, the mainstream entrants account for six out of ten of British-qualified GPs, the somewhat late entrants for three out of ten and the very late entrants for between one and two out of ten.

By contrast, nearly all overseas-qualified GPs are somewhat late or very late entrants to general practice, if one considers the total time spent in the hospital service abroad and in the UK. On that basis, only 5 per cent are mainstream entrants, 21 per cent are somewhat late entrants, and 65 per cent are very late entrants, among whom are 33 per cent who spent upwards of ten years in the hospital service before becoming GPs.

If one considers only the time spent by overseas-qualified GPs in the hospital service in the UK, this is still longer than for British-qualified GPs. On average, overseas-qualified GPs spent 60 months in the hospital service in this country before converting to general practice, compared with 44 months for the British-qualified. This, of course, ignores the time previously spent by the overseas doctors in the hospital service abroad.

Type of health district
One factor that could contribute to the relatively slow progress of overseas-qualified doctors is their concentration in non-teaching districts where opportunities for postgraduate training are still likely to be poorer than in teaching districts in spite of efforts to raise standards in the less favoured areas. We saw in Chapter II that only 19 per cent of overseas-qualified hospital doctors (excluding white anglophones) are working in a teaching district or London postgraduate hospital, compared with 45 per cent of British-qualified hospital doctors and a similar proportion of white anglophones (47 per cent). It is important to establish whether overseas-qualified doctors, purely by virtue of being overseas-qualified, are less likely to be able to find a job in a teaching district, or whether their chances are lower for some other reason, for example because of imperfect English, because they are less well qualified at the postgraduate level or because opportunities are fewer in teaching districts in the specialties which they wish to pursue.

The age distributions of British and overseas-qualified doctors are, of course, markedly different, but this does not account for the different distribution across teaching and non-teaching districts, which contain similar proportions of doctors within the various age groups. Because of a special training system for senior registrars, a high proportion of doctors in this grade are within teaching districts: thus 84 per cent of senior registrars are in teaching districts compared with 34 per cent of hospital doctors in other grades. Within the senior registrar grade, the difference between British and overseas-qualified doctors is comparatively small: 88 per cent of British-qualified senior registrars are in teaching districts compared with 74 per cent of overseas-qualified senior registrars. Within each of the other grades, however, the differences are wide. Thus, 47 per cent of British-qualified senior house officers are in teaching districts compared with 15 per cent of overseas-qualified SHOs. The parallel figures for registrars are 54 per cent compared with 21 per cent, and for medical assistants and consultants they are 36 per cent compared with 17 per cent (Table A23). This shows that overseas-qualified doctors who reach senior registrar grade generally find a job in a teaching district, and do so only slightly less frequently than British-qualified doctors who reach this grade, but that generally speaking the gap between British and overseas-qualified doctors in terms of the numbers working in teaching districts is hardly at all explained by their different levels of seniority.

The distribution across specialties is also largely irrelevant to this issue (Table A24). Within every specialty for which our numbers are adequate for separate analysis a markedly higher proportion of British than of overseas-qualified doctors are working in teaching districts. The gap is narrowest in the case of general medicine and widest in the case of general surgery. In fact, in this latter specialty we find that 46 per cent of British-qualified doctors compared with only 5 per cent of overseas-qualified doctors are working in a teaching district. An overseas doctor has a very small chance indeed of finding a job in general surgery in a teaching district.

There is a marked relationship here with the language test score (Table A25). Overseas-qualified hospital doctors with low scores (0-18) are about half as likely to be working in a teaching district as those with middling or high scores. Some of the difference between British and overseas-qualified doctors in their ability to find jobs in teaching districts can therefore be attributed to a difference in language competence, but by no means all. If we confine the comparison to high scoring hospital doctors (those with scores of 26-29) we find that 47 per cent of the British-qualified compared with 28 per cent of the overseas-qualified are working in teaching districts. The parallel figures for those scoring between 19 and 25 are 38 per cent for the British-qualified and 25 per cent for the overseas-qualified.

One of the purposes of finding a good training job in a teaching district is to enable a doctor to gain the training and experience which will enable him to acquire postgraduate qualifications. Nevertheless, those who have already obtained some postgraduate qualifications may be better placed to get a job in a teaching district than those who have not. Since British doctors are more likely to have postgraduate qualifications than overseas doctors, this might account for the difference between the two groups. However, this kind of explanation seems to carry no weight at all. Thus, among hospital doctors having membership or fellowship, 49 per cent of the British-qualified compared with 29 per cent of the overseas-qualified are working in teaching districts (Table A26), and in the case of those with Part 1 only (who are presumably in particular need of further training and experience to pass the clinically-oriented part 2) the contrast is even stronger (52 per cent compared with 15 per cent).

The conclusion from these detailed analyses is that overseas-qualified doctors are substantially at a disadvantage compared with British-qualified ones in obtaining a job in a teaching district and that the contrast cannot be explained by other factors, except to some extent by a difference in linguistic competence. Although this factor has some importance, overseas doctors whose English is good are nevertheless at a substantial disadvantage in finding a job in a teaching district. This may well be a contributory cause of the relatively slow career and training progress of overseas-qualified doctors.

The present position of British and overseas-qualified doctors compared
Our analysis so far of career progress has shown that overseas doctors lose time and seniority when they come to this country, and that they do not, as a group, subsequently catch up. In fact, there is among them a sub-group which slips further behind. However, it was not possible, when tracing each stage of the career history, to allow for the effects of differences between British and overseas-qualified doctors, for example, in terms of language competence, which might account for some of these differences. In order to estimate the importance of such factors, we shall now pursue a different kind of analysis. Forgetting the various steps by which doctors reached their present position, we shall now make detailed comparisons between the present job types, grades and qualification levels of British and overseas-qualified doctors, in order to assess how far the differences are accounted for by the separate or joint effects of factors other than the mere fact of being overseas or British-qualified.

The most basic difference between the two groups lies in the distribution by age. Since doctors from overseas tend to migrate to the UK after working for a period in the country of origin, comparatively few of them are aged 29 or less. Since many of them return to the country of origin after spending up to ten years in the UK, and since much larger numbers have come in the past fifteen years than previously, comparatively few overseas doctors in this country are aged 45 or more, and very few are over the age of 55. Therefore, overseas doctors are concentrated within a middle age range, but on balance tend to be markedly younger than British doctors.

The first step in our analysis must therefore be to compare the job types and grade of British and overseas-qualified doctors within different age groups. First, as regards job type, Table A27 shows that within every age group a smaller proportion of overseas than of British-qualified doctors are GPs, but whereas among doctors aged 30-34 the difference is very large, among those in each of the later age groups it is much smaller. While the great majority of overseas doctors come to the UK to gain training in the hospital service of a kind that is relevant to a specialist career, among those who stay to a later age the proportion who are GPs is not radically different from the proportion of British doctors in the same age groups.

Excluding the GPs, we can now consider the proportion of hospital doctors in each age group who are at the various grades. Among those aged up to 29, the overseas-qualified hospital doctors are in a more senior post than the British-qualified ones. If a finer age analysis were possible, this difference might well disappear, since the overseas-qualified doctors in the age range 23-29 years are distinctly older, on average, than the British-qualified doctors in the same age range.

Within every other age range, the overseas-qualified doctors tend to be in substantially more junior posts than the British-qualified. The most striking single difference is that among hospital doctors aged 35 to 44, 71 per cent of the British-qualified are consultants, compared with only 16 per cent of the overseas-qualified; for those aged 45 to 54, the comparable figures are 87 per cent and 48 per cent, and for those aged 55 or more they are 90 per cent and 54 per cent (Table A27). In fact, nearly half of overseas doctors who have remained in the hospital service in the UK beyond the age of 45 have failed to become consultants.

Thus, the difference in seniority between British and overseas-qualified hospital doctors, while influenced by differences in the age distributions, are by no means explained by them. The point can be expressed more directly by the construction of tables from which the effect of age differences is entirely removed. The first step in such an analysis is to remove doctors in the lowest age range (up to 27) and in the range 55 or more, since the numbers in these two categories among British and overseas-qualified doctors are so widely different as to interfere with any attempt to control for age.

Secondly, the observations can be weighed in such a way that the age profile of both British and overseas-qualified doctors is made to be exactly the same, and identical with the profile of all doctors aged 28-54. This analysis answers the question 'What would the job types and grades of the two groups of doctors be if their age distributions were exactly the same?'. We have carried out this analysis first for all doctors aged 28-54 and secondly for hospital doctors separately.

The first of these analyses shows that, when age is controlled, a higher proportion of British than of overseas-qualified doctors would still be in general practice (55 per cent compared with 30 per cent). The second analysis, comparing the hospital doctors only, shows that British-qualified hospital doctors would still be very much more senior, on average, than overseas-qualified hospital doctors. For example, 49 per cent of the British-qualified would be consultants, compared with only 16 per cent of the overseas-qualified, while only 8 per cent of the British-qualified would be senior house officers, compared with 37 per cent of the overseas-qualified.

These findings show conclusively that, when full allowance is made for differences in age, there is still a wide gap in seniority between British and overseas-qualified doctors. We know, of course, that this is accounted for more by a loss of time and seniority on coming to the UK than by slow progress since coming, although this latter fact is important for a sub-group of overseas doctors.

Table V.13   **Grade of hospital doctors aged 28-54:**
British and overseas-qualified hospital doctors
compared, with age controlled

Column percentages

	British-qualified	Overseas-qualified
House officer	2	1
Senior house officer	8	37
Registrar	22	30
Senior registrar	15	8
Medical assistant	*	4
Consultant	49	16
Not stated	4	4
Base: Hospital doctors aged 28-54 years		
Unweighted	*285*	*640*
Weighted	*1,726*	*1,685*

NB Special weighting has been used in this table to equalise the age profile of the two groups. For explanation, see the text.

We saw in Chapter II that the qualification level of overseas-qualified GPs tends to be higher than that of British GPs, but overseas-qualified hospital doctors are substantially less well qualified than British hospital doctors. This can be seen both as a cause and a consequence of a failure to progress in the hospital service. Again, the difference is influenced by the difference in age profiles, but is by no means explained by it. When we compare British and overseas-qualified hospital doctors within the same age groups according to the highest postgraduate medical qualification that they possess, we still find substantial differences. Among those aged 30-34 it is not, perhaps, surprising to find that a far higher proportion (74 per cent) of the British-qualified than of the overseas-qualified (19 per cent) have obtained membership or fellowship, since at this stage many of the overseas doctors have been in the UK for a comparatively short time. But the differences remain large for the later age groups: thus, among those aged 35-44, 81 per cent of British-qualified hospital doctors have obtained membership or fellowship compared with 43 per cent of the overseas-qualified, and although the differences are reduced for later age groups, they remain substantial. It is important to note (Table A28) that the proportion of overseas-qualified hospital doctors who have obtained membership or fellowship is about the same for those aged 35-44 and for those aged 45-54 (43 per cent and 40 per cent respectively) but substantially lower for those aged 55 or more (21 per cent). This shows that a substantial proportion of those who have stayed in the hospital service beyond the age of about 40 have never achieved the qualification for which most of them come, and among those who have stayed into late middle age, the great majority are failures in this respect. Others, of course, may have succeeded and returned to the country of origin, but among those who stay the failure rate is high.

Allowing for differences in age distributions, we have shown that overseas-qualified doctors tend to have lower qualifications and to be at lower grades than British-qualified doctors. The next step is to consider whether the large difference in grades is explained by the difference in qualification level. Confining our attention to hospital doctors, and not allowing at present for the differences in age distributions, we find that 68 per cent of British doctors with membership or fellowship are consultants, compared with 28 per cent of overseas doctors (Table A29). Reviewing also those with lower qualifications, we find that, generally, overseas-qualified doctors tend to be much more junior than British-qualified doctors with the same qualifications.

Still forgetting, for the time being, the effects of differences in age profiles, we can also allow for the influence of command of English in determining a hospital doctor's grade. Among very high-scoring hospital doctors (those scoring 26-29) there is little difference, in terms of grade, between the British and overseas-qualified. Among those with middling scores (19-25) there is still some difference in seniority, though it is smaller than the differences with which we started: 29 per cent of the British-qualified are consultants compared with 7 per cent of the overseas-qualified. Among low-scoring doctors no comparison can be made, since no significant number of British-qualified doctors achieve low scores.

If these findings are looked at in a different way, it is clear that language test score is very strongly related to grade: overseas-qualified doctors with high scores tend very strongly to be more senior than those with lower scores. Therefore, when comparisons are made between British and overseas-qualified doctors with similar scores, much of the contrast in seniority is removed. This does suggest that command of English is an important factor — more important than a difference in qualification level — in bringing about the contrast in seniority between British and overseas-qualified doctors. However, the effect is overstated by the statistics just quoted, because older overseas doctors tend very strongly to score higher on the language test than younger ones. Thus, when we compare overseas-qualified and British-qualified doctors scoring 26-29, we are comparing a younger British group with an older overseas one, so that the apparent similarity in seniority between the two groups is somewhat misleading.

In fact, language competence, qualification level and seniority are all strongly related to age. Because of this, the tendency for differences between British and overseas doctors to disappear when command of

79

English is controlled may be misleading. Are high-scoring overseas doctors as senior as high-scoring British ones because their English is good, or because they are older?

To answer this key question, we have carried out a final analysis which simultaneously controls for the effects of age, language competence and qualification level. It defines a group of British and overseas-qualified doctors with equivalent qualifications (membership or fellowship of a Royal College) and language competence (at least 21 on the test) and shows what the job types and grades of the two groups would be if their age distributions were exactly the same.

Among this group, a higher proportion of the overseas-qualified than of the British-qualified would be GPs (21 per cent compared with 13 per cent). Looking at the two comparable groups of hospital doctors, we find that 63 per cent of the British-qualified group would be consultants, compared with 38 per cent of the overseas-qualified group; 41 per cent of the overseas-qualified group would be senior house officers or registrars, compared with 18 per cent of the British-qualified group.

Table V.14   Grade of hospital doctors aged 28-54 who have obtained Membership or Fellowship and score 21-29 on the language test, British and overseas qualified doctors compared, with age controlled

Column percentages

	British-qualified	Overseas-qualified
House officer	—	—
Senior house officer	2	7
Registrar	16	34
Senior registrar	18	16
Medical assistant	—	3
Consultant	63	38
Not stated	2	2
Base: British and overseas-qualified doctors controlled for age		
Unweighted	*173*	*113*
Weighted	*773*	*774*

NB Special weighting has been used in this table to equalise the age profiles of the two groups. For explanation, see the text.

We have shown that overseas-qualified doctors tend to have made substantially less career progress than British-qualified doctors after the joint effects of age, qualification level and linguistic competence have been taken into account.

Summary
In the earlier part of this chapter we compared the way that British and overseas doctors evaluate their career experience in relation to their early preferences and objectives. We found that overseas doctors were more likely than British doctors to have become GPs against their inclination, and more likely to be practising in a specialty that was not their first choice. Overseas doctors were found to be concentrated to some extent in the specialties that were not only generally less popular but also less popular among overseas doctors. Overseas doctors were distinctly more likely than British doctors to feel that they had progressed, in terms of postgraduate training and experience, more slowly than they had expected. There was also evidence that they had, in fact, achieved their postgraduate training objectives more slowly, or had a poorer chance of achieving them at all.

In a detailed analysis of actual career progress, we first of all considered the transition of overseas doctors from the country of origin to the UK. We found that they tended to lose time and seniority at this stage, and it seemed that the most important part of the disparity between overseas and British doctors dated from the moment of transition. When considering progress once established in this country, we found that among overseas doctors who did progress, the rate of progress was comparable with that of British doctors, although there was no tendency to catch up. However, there was a sub-group of overseas doctors who tended to get stuck, particularly at SHO level; overseas doctors still in this grade had on average spent twice as long in it as British doctors.

Looking at the career path of GPs, we found that they could be divided into mainstream entrants to general practice (who become GPs within three years of graduation) and later entrants. Whereas four out of ten British GPs were later entrants, nearly all overseas GPs fell into this group. In fact, overseas GPs had spent longer in the hospital service in the UK alone than had British GPs. This, combined with the fact that a relatively high proportion of overseas GPs had passed the membership or fellowship examination, underlines the finding that they had often entered general practice against their inclination.

There was a strong tendency for overseas-qualified hospital doctors to be working in non-teaching districts, and this could help to account for the tendency to progress slowly. The concentration in non-teaching districts was associated to some extent with inadequate English, but not with any other factor. Nevertheless, even among overseas doctors with good English, penetration into the teaching districts was comparatively low.

In the later part of the chapter we tried to account for the wide difference between overseas and British-qualified doctors, in terms of their job types, grades and qualification levels, by relating these variables with each other and with others such as language competence and age. We found that overseas doctors were more junior and less well-qualified than British doctors partly because they were younger, and partly because of imperfect English; and also that they tended to be more junior partly because they were less well-qualified. However, even when the effect of age, qualification level and language competence were all allowed for, there remained a substantial gap in seniority between the two groups. The earlier findings suggest that this is partly, and more importantly, because of slippage at the moment of transition from the home country to the UK, but partly because of slower progress once established in this country.

These findings show that the tendency for overseas doctors to be more dissatisfied with their progress than British doctors is justified by the facts. However, the kind of analysis that we have carried out concentrates on the difference between the two groups. To balance this, it should be remembered that nearly half of overseas doctors have progressed as fast as they expected (compared with three quarters of British doctors), and that in spite of a tendency for overseas doctors to progress more slowly than comparable British doctors, many do achieve their objectives in coming and progress at similar rates to comparable British doctors. Also, there is some evidence that the more successful overseas doctors tend to return quickly to their countries of origin, and if this is so, any survey of the stock of overseas doctors must be biassed, to some extent, towards those who have been less successful and who are more likely to stay. This is, of course, not so much a bias as a fact about the stock of overseas doctors in the NHS, which contains a disproportionately high number of the relatively unsuccessful. It is an important finding for the British health services that among those overseas doctors who have remained in the UK for a long period or permanently there is a high proportion who have failed to achieve their training objectives.

VI Present Experience and Future Plans of Hospital Doctors

From comparing the career histories of British and overseas-qualified doctors, we now go on to consider their present experience and future plans. In the case of hospital doctors, who are the subject of this chapter, we shall focus on the range of experience and opportunities for training provided by the present job, and on the importance of ethnic differences and language problems in the context of day-to-day work. The broader issues connected with the ethnic dimension, such as doctors' views of the competence of overseas doctors and of the fairness of selection procedures, will be considered in a later chapter.

Problems and difficulties

Before any specific questions about their present experience had been asked, hospital doctors were given the opportunity to describe in their own words any problems or difficulties that they had. Just under half of all hospital doctors (46 per cent) said that they had some problems or difficulties in pursuing a career in the hospital service in England; if anything, a slightly higher proportion of the British-qualified (48 per cent) than of the overseas-qualified (42 per cent) felt that they had problems. The problems and difficulties mentioned fall into five major groups. The first and most frequently mentioned is difficulties to do with job opportunities: 26 per cent of all hospital doctors (similar proportions of the British and overseas-qualified) mention difficulties of this kind. The second group of difficulties is those to do with study and training which, perhaps surprisingly, are mentioned more often by British-qualified (17 per cent) than by overseas-qualified hospital doctors (7 per cent). A third type of difficulty, low pay, is mentioned almost exclusively by British-qualified doctors (by 9 per cent compared with 1 per cent of the overseas-qualified). Difficulties in the fourth group, those to do with discrimination, language or ethnic differences, are mentioned comparatively infrequently, but more often by overseas than by British-qualified doctors. Discrimination against coloured people or foreigners is mentioned specifically by six per cent of overseas-qualified doctors at this point in the questionnaire, where the subject has not been raised by the interviewer. The fifth and final group of difficulties mentioned are those that relate to the system (resources, 'the state of the NHS', bureaucracy). These are mentioned almost exclusively by British-qualified doctors, but not very frequently.

It is clear from these findings that overseas-qualified hospital doctors are no more likely than British-qualified ones to feel that they currently face difficulties in pursuing a career in the hospital service, and that the major difficulties, as seen by both groups of doctors, lie in finding suitable jobs with the opportunity for appropriate study and training. Table VI.1 shows that the similarities between the responses of the two groups are more striking than the differences. However, British doctors are more likely than overseas doctors to place an emphasis on a lack of opportunity for study and training, as distinct from job opportunities. They are also far more likely to complain about the level of pay and about what they consider to be shortcomings of the system. On the other hand, overseas doctors are more concerned than British doctors about ethnic differences and language problems. The proportion of overseas doctors who spontaneously mention colour discrimination is, however, small (six per cent) as it was at earlier questions, and this confirms that

Table VI.1   Problems or difficulties as a hospital doctor in England, by country of qualification.

	Total	British-qualified	Overseas-qualified
			Column percentages
Any problems or difficulties			
Yes	46	48	42
No	53	51	57
Don't know	1	*	1
Problems or difficulties encountered			
Job opportunities			
Poor job opportunities	14	13	15
Cannot get job in chosen specialty	5	5	6
Cannot get a good training job/ job at a teaching hospital	4	4	6
Frequent job changes/insecurity	4	4	3
Promotion too slow.	2	3	1
Any mention of job opportunities	26	25	28
Study/Training			
Not enough time for study	8	9	4
Lack of advice/information/ guidance or training opportunity	4	6	1
Lack of training in the jobs I have had	4	5	3
Any mention of study or training	13	17	7

Table VI.1 (cont'd)

	Total	British-qualified	Overseas-qualified
		Column percentages	
Pay			
Pay inadequate/too low	6	9	1
Discrimination, language, ethnic differences			
Discrimination against coloured people or foreigners	3	2	6
Discrimination against women	1	2	*
Language problems	1	*	2
Dissatisfied with (Asian) junior staff	1	1	—
Relationships between ethnic or national groups	*	—	1
The system			
Lack of finance or resources in hospitals	3	3	1
Too much bureaucracy/ inefficient administration	1	2	—
Difficult to maintain standards because of the state of the NHS	1	2	—
Political interference with clinical freedom	1	1	1
Any mention of the system	5	6	1
Other points			
Lack of married accommodation	2	3	2
Failed exams	1	1	1
Relationship with superiors	1	1	1
Other answers	2	2	2
Don't know	1	1	*
Base: All hospital doctors			
Unweighted	*1,251*	*539*	*712*
Weighted	*2,567*	*1,733*	*834*

Q124 Do you feel that you have had any problems or difficulties in pursuing a career in the hospital service in England?
Q125 What problems or difficulties have you had?

the majority of overseas doctors are not quick to put this interpretation on their difficulties.

While British and overseas-qualified hospital doctors do not differ much in the extent and nature of the problems and difficulties which they feel they are currently facing, it remains true, as we saw in the last

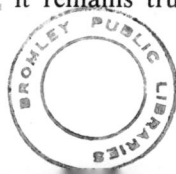

chapter, that overseas doctors are more likely than British doctors to feel that they have progressed slowly towards their objectives over their career in Britain as a whole.

Hours of work
The opportunities for study and training afforded by a hospital job depend on a large number of factors including the range of medical experience provided, the amount and quality of informal teaching and guidance from senior staff, the opportunity to attend courses and seminars inside and outside the hospital, the library and laboratory facilities and the amount of time available for private study. This last factor is a particularly crucial one. Many hospital doctors, particularly those at junior grades, work long hours and are also on call for further lengthy periods. The best training jobs are ones which, while providing intensive experience on the job, do not impose such long hours of work as to make private study impossible.

The average (mean) total hours spent either working or on call during one week was 88 for British-qualified hospital doctors and 90 for the overseas-qualified (Table A32), and the average number of hours spent actually working was 57 for the British-qualified and 61 for the overseas-qualified. The difference in the number of hours 'actually working', though small, might be statistically significant, but when the findings are analysed by the grade of post any such difference disappears. Junior doctors tend to work substantially longer hours than senior ones (Table A33), and this applies to British and overseas doctors equally. Within each particular grade there are no significant differences in the hours worked, or in the total hours spent working and on call, between the two groups of doctors. In this respect it is clear that overseas-qualified hospital doctors are not at a disadvantage.

Analysis by specialty (Table A34) shows that doctors in general surgery, and to a lesser extent, general medicine, tend to work unusually long hours. It is significant that these are the two most popular specialties. The shortest hours are worked by doctors in radiology and radiotherapy, psychiatry and accident and emergency.

Analysis of hours worked by teaching versus non-teaching district shows a paradoxical pattern. Overall the hours worked by doctors in the two types of district are similar, and if anything higher in teaching districts. However, among British doctors hours worked are distinctly higher in teaching than in non-teaching districts (59.6 compared with 54.4) whereas among overseas doctors the opposite is the case (58.4 compared with 62.3). If the figures are compared in a different way, they show that British and overseas doctors in teaching districts work similar hours, whereas in non-teaching districts, overseas doctors work markedly longer hours than British doctors (62.3 compared with 54.4). To the extent that long hours are undesirable, this suggests that within the non-teaching districts, overseas doctors tend to be doing the less desirable jobs.

Opportunity for training and relevant experience

As many answers to open questions show, hospital doctors often discuss junior posts in terms of whether they are 'good training jobs'. Although this way of thinking is understandable in a general way, it is quite difficult to define in concrete terms just what it is that makes a job good from the training point of view. Part of the difficulty is that doctors have in mind an aura of prestige that surrounds certain hospitals or certain specialties within them as well as concrete aspects of the job from day to day. Another difficulty is that much of what a junior doctor gets out of a job depends on informal contacts with senior staff which are difficult to evaluate or quantify.

We nevertheless designed some survey questions which obtain the informant's assessment of the range of experience and opportunity for training and study provided by the job, and then investigated in more detail some of the concrete things and events — such as libraries and contact with senior staff — which may underlie such general assessments. These questions were asked of junior doctors (that is, all except consultants).

Table VI.2   Usefulness of experience from the present job: junior doctors[1] by country of qualification

		Column percentages	
		Qualified in:	
	UK/Eire	White anglophone country	Elsewhere
Very useful	66	48	41
Quite useful	31	52	47
Not very useful	3	—	9
Not useful at all	*	—	2
Don't know	*	—	2
Base: Junior hospital doctors			
Unweighted	*326*	*40*	*583*
Weighted	*903*	*56*	*672*

1 Junior hospital doctors are all except consultants.

Q141 In terms of its range and balance, how useful is the experience that you are getting from this job?

Two general assessments were obtained, one of the medical experience provided, the other of the opportunities for study. From the first of these we find that the great majority of junior doctors, whatever their country of qualification, believe that their present job provides very useful or quite useful experience. However, there is a small, but definite, difference here between the assessments of British and overseas-qualified doctors. Thus, 66 per cent of British doctors said that the job provided very useful experience, compared with 48 per cent of white anglophones and 41 per cent of other overseas-qualified doctors. This difference remains when comparisons are made within particular grades of post, and at SHO level the contrast is stronger. We found that 62 per cent of British-qualified SHOs considered that their job provided very useful experience, compared with 35 per cent of overseas-qualified SHOs. It may be significant that the SHO level is the one at which a proportion of overseas doctors seem to get stuck. Doctors in the less popular specialties tend to find their experience less useful, and this is certainly related to the difference between British and overseas doctors; the most striking example is that only 22 per cent of junior doctors in geriatrics (most of whom are overseas-qualified) have found their present experience useful. Analysis by type of district shows no differences between doctors in teaching and non-teaching districts other than those which are a function of the different balance between British and overseas doctors in the two types of area.

Table VI.3 Opinion of opportunities for study in the present job: junior doctors[1] by country of qualification (Q149)

	British-qualified	Overseas-qualified
		Column percentages
Excellent	13	10
Quite good	49	49
Rather poor	24	27
Very poor	12	10
Don't know	2	3
Base: Junior hospital doctors		
Unweighted	*326*	*623*
Weighted	*903*	*729*

1 See footnote (1) on Table VI.2

From the second general assessment we found that junior doctors are less satisfied with opportunities for study than with the range of experience available. Only 12 per cent give the top rating (excellent), half give the second rating (quite good), while one-quarter considered study opportunities to be rather poor and 11 per cent said they are very poor. Here, as Table VI. 3 shows, the ratings given by British and overseas doctors are almost identical. Differences between the ratings given by doctors in various specialties are not very striking, although it is interesting that those in general surgery gave rather low ratings and those in psychiatry rather high ones. This is probably because surgeons tend to work longer hours than psychiatrists. British-qualified doctors in teaching districts are slightly more likely than those in non-teaching districts to think that study opportunities are excellent or quite good (68 per cent compared with 55 per cent) but there is no similar difference in the case of overseas-qualified doctors.

We would not attach great weight to the absolute levels of these ratings because people tend to identify with their jobs to an extent that makes it difficult for them to criticise them strongly. It would be wrong to conclude that most junior hospital jobs are 'good training jobs' or that shortcomings are few. However, the findings do suggest first that there is more dissatisfaction with the study opportunities than with the range of medical experience provided by junior hospital jobs, and secondly that there is no great difference in the level of satisfaction of British and overseas-qualified doctors in either respect. This latter finding contrasts in an interesting way with the earlier one that a much higher proportion of British than of overseas doctors are in teaching districts. Further, we found that junior doctors in teaching districts were hardly more likely than those in non-teaching districts to give higher ratings to the study opportunities or range of experience provided by their jobs. This suggests that jobs in teaching districts may have extrinsic rather than intrinsic advantages: that is, they may not in fact, provide significantly better experience or opportunities for study, but they do carry higher prestige, so that a doctor who has had experience in a teaching district will tend to progress more quickly afterwards.

Three further questions were asked to test the range of experience provided by the job. As an indication of the degree of independent responsibility that they are allowed, junior doctors were asked how often they wrote correspondence and patients' notes. Three-quarters of junior doctors said that they did so regularly, and here there was no significant difference between British and overseas-qualified doctors.

A second indicator is the number of beds for which the doctor is responsible. (Formally, only consultants are responsible for beds, but in practice most junior doctors consider that responsibility for a certain number of beds has been delegated to them.) We found that British-qualified junior doctors were, on average, responsible for 26 beds and overseas-qualified junior doctors for 35. These results suggest that overseas-qualified junior doctors have at least as much delegated authority as the British-qualified, and possibly a heavier workload. The difference between the two groups is partly a consequence of the different distribution across specialties. In addition, we did find in this case a significant difference between teaching and non-teaching districts. Junior doctors in non-teaching districts are responsible, on average, for 33 beds, compared with 25 beds for those in teaching districts, and the differences by type of district remain when British and overseas doctors are considered separately, though they are strongest among overseas doctors. The differences imply that staffing ratios are more favourable in teaching districts. Overseas doctors, because they are concentrated in non-teaching districts, are likely to be responsible for more beds than British doctors.

Table VI.4   Number of beds for which the doctor is responsible: junior doctors by country of qualification, grade and type of district (Q138)

	British-qualified	Overseas-qualified
Grade		
House officer	28.1	n.a.
Senior house officer	26.3	31.0
Registrar	29.4	40.1
Senior registrar	17.5	31.2
Medical assistant	n.a.	n.a.
Type of district		
Teaching district and London		
postgraduate teaching hospital	24.2	26.5
Non-teaching district	27.9	36.9
All junior grades	25.9	34.5

NB The figures given are means. The base for each cell in the table is different.

A third measure of the range of experience provided by a job is the extent to which doctors deal with each of six broadly defined types of case (see Q139). On average, junior doctors said that they regularly dealt with 4½ out of the six types of case, and there is no significant difference here between the British and overseas-qualified. Nine out of ten doctors in both groups said that they regularly dealt with acute cases. The proportion of overseas doctors who regularly dealt with chronic cases was just slightly higher (67 per cent) than for British doctors (61 per cent).

A second series of detailed questions relates to opportunities for study. We found (Table A35) no difference between British and overseas-qualified junior doctors in the number of mornings or afternoons which they are allowed off work for private or formal study (the average is 2.3 in a four-week period). Nor was there any difference in the proportion who have access to adequate library facilities at the hospital (72 per cent of all junior doctors) or elsewhere (a further 19 per cent). In every hospital there should be a consultant, designated the postgraduate tutor, who is responsible for co-ordinating courses and seminars inside the hospital, for providing information about suitable courses elsewhere, and for advising junior doctors on matters connected with postgraduate training. This system is not universally effective, since 28 per cent of junior doctors did not know their postgraduate tutor. However, the proportion in ignorance is exactly the same for the British and overseas-qualified (Table A36). Junior doctors generally spend little time with the postgraduate tutor but overseas-qualified doctors are more likely to spend time with the tutor than British-qualified doctors (30 per cent compared with 15 per cent). Only 30 per cent of junior doctors said that they had access to laboratory facilities for their own research. This proportion was slightly higher among the British-qualified (34 per cent) than among the overseas-qualified (26 per cent). There is a striking difference, in this respect, between teaching and non-teaching districts: 46 per cent of junior doctors in teaching districts have access to laboratories for research, compared with 20 per cent of those in non-teaching districts, and it is this contrast that accounts for the difference between British and overseas-qualified doctors. In the area of research and laboratory facilities, we found for the first time an important and substantial intrinsic difference between the two types of district. Finally, we have a measure of the number of hours spent per week in organised study, such as lectures, seminars and study meetings (Table A37). Among all junior doctors, the mean number of hours spent per week was 2.3; 19 per cent spent no time in organised study. Differences between British and overseas-qualified doctors in this respect were slight. A larger proportion of overseas than of British doctors spent no time in organised study (27 per cent compared with 14 per cent), and those who did take part in organised study among the British-qualified tended to put in more hours than the overseas-qualified, so that the mean number of hours spent by the British was rather higher (2.5 compared with 2.1). There was no difference between doctors in teaching and non-teaching districts.

In short, on the basis of the admittedly rather crude meaures available to us, we can find few differences between British and overseas-qualifed doctors in terms of the range of experience or study opportunities currently available to them, and the differences that do appear are small. This remains true whether we rely on junior doctors' general assessments or on more concrete facts about working and training. Except in access to laboratory facilities for research, differences between teaching and non-teaching districts are also surprisingly small.

Working relationships

A junior doctor is heavily dependent on his consultant in several ways. The consultant is in a position to decide which patients he should see, and what degree of independent responsibility he should take for them. Informal training on the job, perhaps the most important aspect of a junior doctor's training, comes mainly from the consultant, and the amount and quality of informal training will depend on the standard of the particular consultant, his interest in the junior doctor, and the relationship between them. The junior doctor's future job prospects will critically depend on the reference given by his consultant when he seeks a fresh job. Unfortunately, it is not possible within a large scale survey to obtain very sensitive measures of the quality of a junior doctor's relationship with his consultant, partly because the quality of a relationship is an elusive thing, and partly because junior doctors will be reluctant to make criticisms to an outsider of the person on whom they most depend.

The best that we could do was to ask junior doctors to rate their working relationships with their consultants on a scale running from 'excellent' to 'poor' (the scale was intentionally weighted towards the positive end so as to discriminate between very favourable and slightly less favourable responses). As expected, the great majority of junior doctors rated the relationship as 'excellent' (47 per cent) or 'good' (41 per cent); only 9 per cent gave the neutral rating 'acceptable' and a mere 1 per cent the negative rating 'poor'. The ratings of both British and overseas doctors were very favourable, but those of overseas doctors were still more favourable than those of British doctors: thus, 56 per cent of overseas-qualified junior doctors rated the relationship as 'excellent' compared with 40 per cent of British-qualified junior doctors. We do not regard this as conclusive evidence of what actually happens between junior doctors and their consultants, but it does show that overseas-qualified junior doctors are rather less likely than the British-qualified to express complaints on this score.

Naturally, the great majority of junior doctors (90 per cent) have British consultants, but it is interesting that there is some tendency towards ethnic polarisation in a broad sense: that is, a larger proportion of British-qualified junior doctors (94 per cent) than of the overseas-qualified (86 per cent) have British consultants. The ratings of the quality of the relationship with the consultant are not, however, related to the consultant's country of origin.

In order to assess the extent of social mixing between ethnic groups in the hospital, all hospital doctors were asked the question: 'When they are in the hospital but not actually at work, do doctors belonging to different ethnic groups tend to mix together freely or do they tend to remain in separate groups?'. Just over half of hospital doctors (54 per cent) thought the groups mixed together freely, and 35 per cent that they remained in separate groups; the remaining 11 per cent had no definite opinion. Overseas doctors were more likely to think that there was free mixing (62 per cent) than British doctors (50 per cent). These findings show that a substantial minority of both British and overseas doctors think there is little social contact between different ethnic groups in the hospital outside the wards: this may be a potential or actual source of tension.

More directly, all hospital doctors were asked: 'Are there any difficulties or shortcomings in working relationships between coloured and white doctors in this hospital?', and if they answered 'yes' they were asked to describe these difficulties in detail. A majority of both British and overseas doctors said that there were no difficulties or shortcomings of this kind, but British-qualified doctors were markedly more likely to think that there were shortcomings (32 per cent) than anglophones (19 per cent) or other overseas doctors (10 per cent). The difficulties mentioned by overseas doctors other than anglophones are almost exclusively to do with communication, language and culture, though prejudice against overseas doctors on the part of British doctors is mentioned by 2 per cent. In addition to difficulties of communication, language and culture, the anglophones mention variable or low standards among overseas doctors (12 per cent). However, most of the interest here centres on the answers of British doctors, who are substantially more likely to believe that difficulties exist, and who also mention a wider range of difficulties.

Table VI.5   Difficulties in working relationships between white and coloured doctors, by country of qualification

Column percentages

	UK/Eire	White anglophone	Elsewhere
Difficulties or shortcomings			
Yes	32	19	10
No	62	79	87
Don't know	5	2	3
Difficulties:			
Communication, language, culture			
Failure of communication because of language difficulties/inadequate English of overseas doctors	22	6	1
Failure of communication because of cultural differences	4	2	1
Cultural differences leading to hostility/difficulty in forming workable relationships	5	4	2
Different attitudes and assumptions about pain/value of human life/ types of care/behaviour towards patients	4	2	*
Lack of social mixing	2	—	2
Diet/strong-smelling food	*	—	*
Any mention of communication, language, culture	27	11	5

Table VI.5 (cont'd)

Column percentages

	Country of qualification:		
	UK/Eire	White anglophone	Elsewhere

Criticisms of overseas doctors

	UK/Eire	White anglophone	Elsewhere
Variability of standards among overseas doctors/some are incompetent/their standards are low	9	12	*
Some British doctors *think* the standards of overseas doctors are low	1	—	1
Overseas doctors have less dedication to work/have too little sense of urgency/tend to be careless	3	—	*
Overseas doctors tend to be aggressive/arrogant/over-confident/don't easily work in a team	1	—	*
Clinical assistants are a nuisance/incompetent	*	—	—
Some happen to be unco-operative (not because they are coloured or from overseas)	*	1	—
Any criticism of overseas doctors	14	13	2

Other difficulties

	UK/Eire	White anglophone	Elsewhere
Overseas doctors cause an imbalance, weaken the profession, because they work in dead-end departments and in poorer specialties	1	—	—
Overseas doctors weaken the profession because they destroy its united front	*	—	—
Don't know	*	1	—
Base: All hospital doctors			
Unweighted	*539*	*60*	*652*
Weighted	*1,733*	*84*	*749*

Q.153 Are there any difficulties or shortcomings in working relationships between white and coloured doctors in this hospital?
Q.154 If yes, what difficulties?

The answers given by British doctors can be divided into three main categories: difficulties to do with communication, language and culture, which are most frequently mentioned (by 27 per cent): criticisms of

94

overseas doctors, which are fairly common (14 per cent): and references to prejudice against overseas doctors, which are rather rare (2 per cent).

Under the heading of communication, language and culture, 22 per cent of British doctors say that there is a failure of communication specifically because of language difficulties, and a further 4 per cent because of cultural differences. In addition, 5 per cent of British doctors feel that cultural differences lead to hostility or to difficulty in forming working relationships. A small proportion of British doctors (4 per cent) also drew attention to cultural differences as they affect medical practice: the general thrust of these comments is that overseas doctors (that is, Asian doctors, in this context) tend to have a fatalistic attitude towards pain and suffering, put a lower value on human life, and expect patients to be deferential.

Under the heading of criticisms of overseas doctors, 9 per cent of British doctors said that the standards of overseas doctors were low or variable: among these, some went as far as to say that some overseas doctors were incompetent. A further 3 per cent said that overseas doctors had too little dedication to work or sense of urgency. A very small proportion (1 per cent) said that overseas doctors tend to be aggressive or arrogant; this fits in with the idea that Asian doctors expect patients to put up with pain and to be deferential, but relates, in addition, to working relationships with other doctors.

It is important to emphasise, however, that a clear majority of both British and overseas-qualified hospital doctors said that there were no difficulties or shortcomings in working relationships between ethnic groups; at the same time, the receiving group is far more likely to see difficulties than the incoming group.

Language difficulties
Hospital doctors were asked a series of questions about the importance of language difficulties first, in their relationships with other doctors and secondly, in their relationships with patients. The general thrust of the findings is that a substantial proportion of British doctors think that the inadequate English of overseas doctors and of patients belonging to minority groups leads to problems in communication. Few overseas doctors think that they have language difficulties of any kind, and where they do think they have difficulties, they are thinking of the inadequacy of other people's English and not of their own. British doctors may exaggerate the difficulties and overseas doctors may under-estimate them (because they are reluctant to admit to their own shortcomings). Since we know that an important minority of overseas doctors are at a significant linguistic disadvantage, we have to place more emphasis on a tendency on the part of overseas doctors to under-estimate language difficulties than on a tendency on the part of British doctors to exaggerate them.

In detail, we found that 62 per cent of British hospital doctors thought that there were language difficulties in communicating with other doctors, compared with 35 per cent of white anglophones and only 10 per cent of other overseas-qualified doctors. The difference here between British-qualified doctors and white anglophones is interesting, and may be some measure of a tendency to exaggerate on the part of British doctors. The group with which British doctors claimed to have most difficulty in communicating are Indians (45 per cent), Pakistanis or Bangladeshis (36 per cent) and to a lesser extent Arabs (14 per cent). These are also the groups with which overseas-qualified doctors claim to have language difficulties; only one per cent of overseas-qualified doctors thought that they had language difficulties in communicating with white English-speaking doctors (compared with the 62 per cent of British doctors who claimed that they had such difficulties from the other side of the relationship). However, only 7 per cent of British doctors thought that these problems of communciation were severe; 28 per cent described them as moderate and 25 per cent as slight.

Table VI.6 Language difficulties in communicating with other doctors hospital doctors by country of qualification (Qs 155-157)

Column percentages

	Country of qualification:		
	UK/Eire	White anglophone	Elsewhere
Total having language difficulties	62	35	10
of which			
Severe	7	2	1
Moderate	28	25	6
Slight	25	7	3
Uncertain how serious	2	—	—
Ethnic groups with which most difficulty experienced:			
Indians	45	20	5
Pakistani/Bangladeshi	36	12	3
Middle Eastern/Arab	14	11	3
White English-speaking	*	1	1
Other groups	9	12	1
Uncertain which groups	3	1	*
Base: Hospital doctors			
Unweighted	*539*	*60*	*652*
Weighted	*1,733*	*84*	*749*

More than half of British hospital doctors (56 per cent) said they had language difficulties in communicating with patients; the main ethnic groups mentioned in this connection are Indians (35 per cent), Pakistanis or Bangladeshis (31 per cent) and Continental Europeans (18 per cent).

Again, a smaller proportion of doctors from white anglophone countries
(44 per cent) than of British doctors thought they had language difficulties, although the difference is smaller than in the case of relationships with other doctors. A comparatively small proportion of other
overseas-qualified doctors (19 per cent) thought they had language difficulties, though in this case, an appreciable proportion (8 per cent)
admit to difficulties in communicating with white English patients. The
admission is easier to make in this case, since overseas doctors can
ascribe the difficulties to local accents and dialects rather than to their
own inadequacy. Difficulties in communication with patients are
thought by all groups to occur rarely or perhaps quite often, but are not
generally thought to occur frequently.

**Table VI.7 Language difficulties in communicating with patients:
hospital doctors by country of qualification. (Qs 158-160)**

Column percentages

| | Country of qualification: | | |
	UK/Eire	White anglophone	Elsewhere
Total having language difficulties	56	44	19
of which			
Frequently	7	7	*
Quite often	15	11	3
Rarely	35	26	16
Uncertain how often	—	—	*
Ethnic groups with which difficulty			
most often experienced:			
Indians	35	23	5
Pakistani/Bangladeshi	31	25	5
Europeans	18	11	4
West Indians	5	1	1
White English-speaking	2	5	8
Other groups	13	17	1
Uncertain which groups	1	1	*
Base: Hospital doctors			
Unweighted	*539*	*60*	*652*
Weighted	*1,733*	*84*	*749*

Given that overseas doctors rarely admit to difficulties caused by their
own linguistic inadequacy, it is not surprising to find that their answers
to these questions are not related to the language test score. Even very
low-scoring overseas doctors very seldom believe that they have difficulties in communicating either with other doctors or with patients
because of their own inadequate English. Among British doctors, those
at all grades of hospital post have similar views about language difficulties.

Reaction of patients

It was pointed out in an earlier chapter that most overseas-qualified doctors are 'coloured', that is, they would be perceived as racially distinct from the white majority by patients, most of whom are white. It is important to establish how far racial prejudice on the part of patients or the perception of a cultural difference, is thought to cause a problem for overseas doctors.

This does not seem to be a salient factor, since it was not mentioned spontaneously by overseas doctors when asked about problems or difficulties in pursuing a career in the UK in a general way. However, when the question was specifically raised, we did find that a substantial proportion of doctors thought there was some problem of this kind.

Table VI.8   Reaction of patients to treatment by coloured doctors:
hospital doctors by country of qualification (Qs 161-163)

Column percentages

	Country of qualification:		
	UK/Eire	White anglophone	Elsewhere
Patients dislike being treated by a coloured doctor:	65	54	34
This is:			
Common	5	10	1
Fairly common	18	11	4
Rather uncommon	29	17	15
Rare	11	17	15
Don't know how common	2	—	*
This is a:			
Serious problem	10	4	3
Slight problem	37	33	14
No real problem	15	14	16
Don't know how serious	3	2	1
Base: Hospital doctors			
Unweighted	*539*	*60*	*652*
Weighted	*1,733*	*84*	*749*

All hospital doctors were asked 'In your experience, do English patients ever dislike being treated by a coloured doctor?', and those who answered 'Yes' were further asked how commonly this happened and how serious a problem it was. Among British-qualified doctors, Table VI.8 shows that 65 per cent said that patients do sometimes dislike being treated by a coloured doctor; comparatively few (5 per cent) thought this was common, but 18 per cent thought it was fairly common, while 40 per cent thought it rather uncommon or rare. As many as 10 per cent of

British doctors thought that patients' antipathy to coloured doctors was a serious problem, 37 per cent thought it was a slight problem, while the remainder thought that it was no real problem. The responses of white anglophone doctors are fairly similar to those of British doctors, although they tend to emphasise this issue rather less. Overseas-qualified doctors, on the other hand, towards whom the antipathy is supposed to be directed, are much less aware of a problem than British doctors, as the figures in Table VI.8 indicate. It is possible that British doctors tend to exaggerate a difficulty connected with overseas doctors, whereas overseas doctors themselves tend to under-estimate it, although we cannot judge how much weight to attach to each of these factors. Certainly, appreciable proportions of both groups of doctors thought that patient resistance to coloured doctors was a problem, although from the answers to open question, it is not something at the forefront of their minds.

Future settlement plans

Just over half (58 per cent) of overseas-qualified hospital doctors in England at the time of the survey said that they intended to leave the country in the foreseeable future, generally within two or three years. This means that the population of overseas-qualified hospital doctors falls roughly into two halves: one half consists of doctors who have permanently settled in the UK, while the other half consists of doctors who intend to leave within a comparatively short period. Most of those who intend to leave (81 per cent) intend to return to the country of origin; the remainder intend to move on to one of a wide range of countries, among which Australia and the USA are the most commonly mentioned.

Analysis of intention to leave by year of coming to this country (Figure 1) shows that among overseas-qualified hospital doctors who came to the UK very recently (within the past two years) about three-quarters intend to leave again in the future, whereas among those who came ten or more years ago the great majority intend to remain in the UK. Thus, a majority of the inflow of migrants intend to leave again and actually do so. Among those who have been in this country for a considerable time a majority intend to stay, because they belong to cohorts from which the short stayers have already left. The steepest fall in intention to leave shown by the graph is between doctors who came to the UK in 1971 compared with 1967. This may imply that the commonest actual length of stay is between six and ten years.

We can gain some indication of how intentions to stay or leave change over a stay in the UK by comparing the original intentions of migrants on coming to this country with their present intentions. In an earlier chapter we have shown that 82 per cent of adult migrants originally intended to stay for a period which they could definitely estimate, and a further 11 per cent did not intend to stay permanently, though they could not set a limit to the expected length of their stay. When we analysed the expected

FIGURE 1 **Proportion of overseas hospital doctors who intend to leave the UK in future, by year of coming to the UK**

Per cent who intend to
leave the UK in future

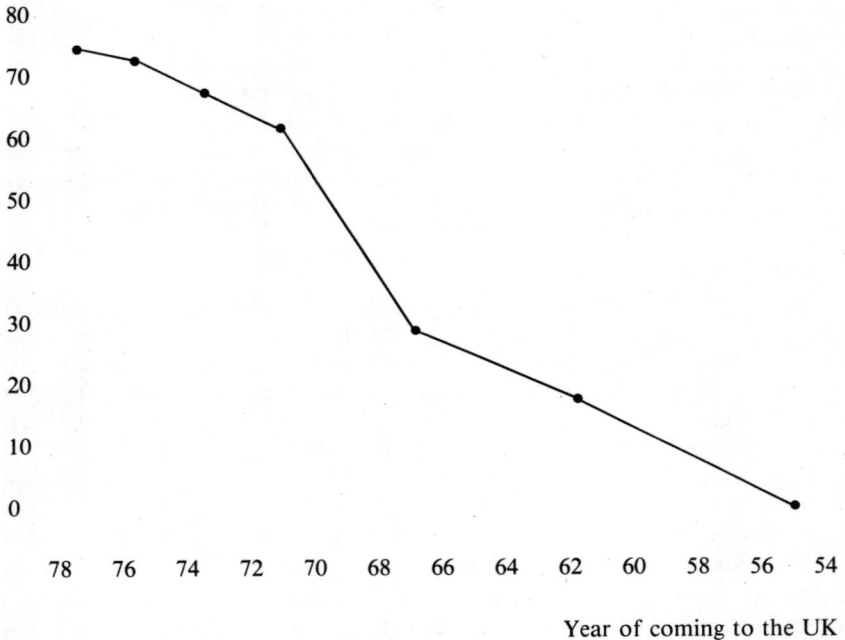

Year of coming to the UK

NB Only hospital doctors who were both born overseas and qualified overseas are included in the graph

length of stay by the actual length of stay to date, we found that most of the earlier migrants who were still here had already stayed for substantially longer than they originally intended. A substantial minority of those who had stayed for longer than they expected to had done so because they had failed to achieve their objectives in the expected time, and the remainder because of the positive attractions of a career in the UK or because they had acquired new links with this country, for example, through marriage.

The present intentions are compared with the original intentions in Table VI.9. Among the earlier migrants, there has been a radical shift from an original intention to leave the UK after a period to present intention to stay for the foreseeable future.

Table VI. 9 Original and present intention[1] to stay in the UK by year of migration (Qs 33, 34 and 126)

Column percentages

	Total	Year of coming to the UK:						
		Up to 1959	1960-1964	1965-1969	1970-1972	1973-1974	1975-1976	1977-1978
Original intention:								
To stay permanently	5	15	2	13	3	2	2	5
To stay indefinitely	11	34	13	7	15	12	3	12
Total intending to stay permanently or indefinitely[2]	16	49	15	20	18	14	5	17
Present intention:								
To stay for foreseeable future	37	94	75	58	30	26	22	23

1 The percentages for 'original intention' are based on adult migrants who are now hospital doctors, while those for 'present intention' are based on all migrants who are now hospital doctors, but this discrepancy between the two groups is not large and has little, if any, effect on the comparison.
2 For the exact wording of the questions, see the questionnaire. 'Stay indefinitely' means did not intend to stay permanently but set no limit to the length of stay. Hence, the proportions who originally intended to stay permanently or indefinitely can be compared with the proportions now intending to stay for the foreseeable future.

For example, among hospital doctors who came between 1960 and 1964, only 15 per cent originally intended to stay permanently or indefinitely, whereas 75 per cent now intend to stay indefinitely. As would be expected, the gap becomes narrower among more recent migrants, but the interesting point is that it does not entirely disappear. Thus, among those who came in 1975 and 1976, only 5 per cent originally intended to stay here permanently or indefinitely, whereas 22 per cent intended to do so at the time of the interview about two years after their arrival. Over the two-year period since their arrival, these doctors have not yet had time to find that they are unable to achieve their objectives. This implies that some migrants do tend to modify their intentions towards staying in this country soon after they arrive because of the positive benefits of pursuing a career here rather than because of difficulties in achieving their objectives.

Among British-qualified hospital doctors there is a significant proportion (18 per cent) who intend to leave the country in the foreseeable future. However, it should not be assumed that all of these British-qualified doctors, if they do follow their intentions, will be permanently lost to the NHS. Among British-qualified doctors generally (including hospital doctors and GPs) we find that 19 per cent have worked abroad in the past, and the median period worked abroad among this group is

101

only 25 months. Taken together these findings are consistent with the theory that most of those British doctors who go to work abroad, return after only a few years. When asked their reasons for wishing to leave the UK in future (Table A39), a substantial proportion of British doctors who intend to leave (40 per cent) explicitly said that they wished to gain experience of medicine in other countries, rather than to settle abroad. The others mentioned either the advantages of pursuing a career abroad or the disadvantages of working in the NHS. Eighteen per cent gave higher rates of pay abroad as a reason for moving, and in addition 17 per cent mentioned poor financial incentives in the UK, relating this either to the NHS pay structure or to the taxation system. Twenty-one per cent referred to 'the state of the NHS', sometimes further characterised as a lack of finance and resources, and 6 per cent to the 'socialist attitude to medicine' as exemplified by the phasing out of private beds, or in a more general lack of reward for merit and enterprise. A wide range of intended destinations were mentioned (Table A38), among which Australia (15 per cent) and the USA (13 per cent) were the most popular.

Among overseas-qualified hospital doctors who intend to leave the UK in future (Table A39), this is generally the confirmation of their original intention. When asked why they intend to leave, 36 per cent specifically referred to their original intention to come to this country for a limited period of training, and over half mentioned the links with the home country which weigh against a permanent migration. In this context, there were no references to difficulties faced by overseas doctors specifically in progressing within the NHS.

From direct questioning we find that overseas-qualified doctors most commonly intend to leave after reaching registrar (62 per cent) or senior registrar level (19 per cent), and only rarely after becoming consultants (6 per cent). This finding can be indirectly confirmed through an analysis of present intentions by present grade (Table A40). Among those at registrar level or below, 71 per cent intend to leave the UK in future, compared with 16 per cent of those at senior registrar level or above. It is roughly correct to regard overseas doctors at the junior grades (registrar and below) as a floating population, and those at the more senior grades (senior registrar and above) as mostly permanently settled in the UK.

In an earlier chapter we found that it was the prime objective of a majority of migrants to pass the membership or fellowship examination before leaving the UK (in fact, 77 per cent of those who originally intended to leave after a period meant to obtain membership or fellowship first). Looking now at present intentions, we find that 69 per cent of overseas-qualified hospital doctors who intend to leave in future either have membership or fellowship already, or still intend to get it before leaving. This shows that doctors who still intend to leave do not set their sights lower after a period in this country. However, we know from findings already presented that there is a significant group who originally intended to leave after a period, but who have now decided to stay after failing to get the expected qualifications.

Type of career planned
Because the balance of supply and demand varies between specialties, hospital doctors often have to settle for a specialty that was not their first choice, and this applies to a higher proportion of overseas than of British-qualified doctors. However, most doctors in both groups have now reconciled themselves to remaining in their present specialty, and overseas doctors have generally come to terms with the opportunities available to them (as have British doctors); only 8 per cent of overseas-qualified hospital doctors and 11 per cent of the British-qualified now intend to change to a different specialty (Table VI.10).

Table VI.10 Future career plans of British and overseas-qualified hospital doctors (Qs. 133 and 134)

		Column percentages
	British-qualified	Overseas-qualified
Intend to:		
Remain in this specialty	77	86
Change to a different specialty	11	8
Change to general practice	6	3
Change to another medical career	5	2
Don't know	1	1
Base: Hospital doctors		
Unweighted	*539*	*712*
Weighted	*1,733*	*834*

Overall, the proportion of both groups who intend to go into general practice is very small (6 per cent of the British-qualified and 3 per cent of the overseas-qualified). Even among house officers and senior house officers, the proportion is still relatively small (19 per cent of the British-qualified and 5 per cent of the overseas-qualified). It is quite clear from this that a substantial proportion of present house officers and senior house officers who now intend to pursue a hospital career will later convert to general practice. Nearly half (49 per cent) of British-qualified doctors are GPs, yet only 15 per cent of British-qualified house officers and 21 per cent of senior house officers intend to become GPs. Although fewer overseas-qualified doctors are destined to become GPs, there is a similar gap between preferences of the most junior and the likely outcomes. This confirms the assumption made in our earlier analysis of the career paths of GPs that late entrants to general practice, who form an important proportion of the total, are also reluctant entrants.

VII The Present Experience of General Practitioners

The great majority of overseas-qualified doctors originally intended to be hospital specialists, and came to the UK to obtain specialised training and experience to this end, in most cases intending to return home after a period. However, some overseas doctors have decided to stay in the UK as GPs, often after having passed the membership or fellowship examinations. These doctors, who are nearly all late or very late entrants to general practice, accounted for one-quarter of overseas-qualified doctors in the NHS at the time of the survey. Among British-qualified doctors at the time of the survey, nearly one half of the total were general practitioners, and although a substantial proportion of these were late entrants to general practice, there is also a substantial proportion who originally intended to be GPs and who entered general practice after only two or three years in the hospital service. British and overseas-qualified GPs are therefore somewhat contrasting groups. The purpose in this chapter is to compare their present experience in order to assess whether overseas-qualified GPs tend to be dissatisfied with a branch of the profession which they have generally chosen at a relatively late stage and often reluctantly, to see whether they tend to have different and possibly less desirable kinds of practice from British GPs, and to assess how far the two groups are providing a comparable service to their patients.

Problems and difficulties
Before they had been asked any questions about specific aspects of their present experience, GPs were asked the general question "Do you feel that you have had any problems or difficulties in practising as a GP in England?, and if they answered 'Yes' they were asked to describe these problems in their own words. We found that consciousness of problems and difficulties was much higher among British than among overseas-qualified GPs; 52 per cent of British compared with 25 per cent of overseas-qualified GPs said they had any problems or difficulties. Table VII.1 shows that the commonest complaints among British-qualified GPs were ones relating to the system: 29 per cent made some complaint of this kind, and 20 per cent specifically said that the NHS is inefficient or frustrating. By contrast, overseas-qualified GPs rarely made com-

plaints of this kind and this accounts for a substantial part of the difference in the proportion of each group who are conscious of any problems. The two other chief causes of complaint among British GPs are pay and hours of work.

Table VII.1 Problems and difficulties of GPs

Column percentages

	British-qualified	Overseas-qualified
Experience of problems or difficulties:		
Yes	52	25
No	48	75
Don't know	1	—
Kind of problems:		
Pay		
Inadequate pay (in early years as GP)	11	4
Payment structure does not encourage good care/lack of incentive	7	*
Any mention of pay	17	4
Hours		
Always/very often on call	8	2
Problem of combining practice with family commitments/children	3	3
Any mention of hours	11	5
Relationships		
With local GPs	3	2
With hospital staff	1	*
Any mention of relationships	4	3
The system		
The NHS is inefficient/frustrating	20	4
The NHS is inflexible/does not respond quickly to new developments in medicine and care	3	—
Access to hospital facilities	11	2
Nature of the area: decaying/inner city/ poor environment	1	*
Any mention of the system	29	4
Other answers	10	13
Don't know	*	*
Base: All GPs		
Unweighted	*477*	*253*
Weighted	*1,649*	*274*

Q.94 Do you feel that you have had any problems or difficulties in practising as a GP in England?
Q.95 What problems have you had?

These findings certainly show that active discontent is more common among British than among overseas-qualified doctors, but this is probably because of a difference in expectations and reference points rather than a difference in actual experience. For example, the overseas GPs are unlikely to complain about the NHS as a system probably because it is better than the other systems that they know about (in the countries of origin), whereas among British GPs the NHS is tacitly compared to some notion of private medical services as they might be organised. The reference points of the two groups with regard to pay may also be different: the overseas-qualified GPs may still tacitly make comparisons with pay in the home country, whereas the British GPs may compare themselves with specialists in Britain, or with GPs in the USA.

The problems and difficulties mentioned by both groups are ones arising from causes external to themselves. In line with this, no overseas-qualified GPs said that they had difficulties in communicating with patients or with other doctors because of language difficulties or cultural differences.

Practices in conurbations are sometimes said to be demanding and unpopular. However, GPs in the conurbations are no more likely to mention problems and difficulties than those elsewhere, and the difficulties mentioned by GPs in the two broad types of area follow the same pattern. This is also true of British and of overseas-qualified GPs considered separately from each other. The differences in the answers given are related strongly to the country of qualification, and not at all to the type of area where the practice is.

In general there is no evidence either among British or among overseas-qualified GPs, that late entrants to general practice are more likely to have complaints than mainstream entrants. However, overseas-qualified GPs who have passed the membership or fellowship examinations (and who therefore had good prospects, prima facie, of pursuing a successful career in the hospital service) are more likely than those without this qualification to express complaints (41 per cent of those with membership or fellowship compared with 21 per cent of other overseas-qualified GPs).

Among British-qualified GPs, men are more likely to have complaints than women (54 per cent compared with 38 per cent) and men's complaints are much more likely to be directed towards the system; for example, 22 per cent of the men complain about the inefficiency of the NHS compared with 4 per cent of the women. Although more women than men say that they have difficulties in combining general practice with family commitments, only a small proportion of women mention difficulties of this kind (9 per cent of the British-qualified and 13 per cent of the overseas-qualified).

Preference for general practice

Since we know that a substantial proportion of GPs, especially among the overseas-qualified, have chosen general practice at a late stage and often reluctantly, it is important to assess how far they are reconciled to this career. After many detailed questions about their present job had been asked, as a summation of their attitude GPs were asked 'Would you prefer to be a hospital doctor rather than a GP?', and they were then asked to give the reasons for their answer in their own words. Only 7 per cent of the British-qualified, compared with 30 per cent of the overseas-qualified, said they would prefer to be hospital doctors. This attitude is strongly related to the stage at which doctors entered general practice. Among overseas-qualified GPs who entered general practice after six years or less in the hospital service, only 11 per cent said they would prefer to be hospital doctors, compared with 50 per cent of those who previously spent 10 years or more in the hospital service (Table VII.2). The same relationship appears to exist among British-qualified doctors, although it cannot be demonstrated so clearly because there are too few very late entrants to general practice.

Table VII.2   Whether GPs would prefer to be hospital doctors: various analyses (Q.114)

	Per cent of each group who would prefer to be hospital doctors	Base:	
		Unweighted	Weighted
All GPs	11	730	1923
British-qualified	7	477	1649
Overseas-qualified	30	253	274
British-qualified			
Time spent as hospital doctor:			
1-18 months	5	102	372
19-36 months	8	118	423
3-6 years	8	138	489
Over 6 years	10	82	254
Time spent as GP:			
Up to 5 years	13	65	241
5-13 years	8	88	299
13-23 years	10	157	547
23-33 years	1	101	347
Over 33 years	5	34	115
Overseas-qualified			
Time spent as hospital doctor:			
Up to 6 years	11	61	71
6-10 years	30	80	84
Over 10 years	50	82	86
Time spent as GP:			
Up to 5 years	41	85	86
5-13 years	31	103	113
Over 13 years	13	39	46

The reasons most commonly given by GPs for preferring a career in the hospital service are that they have specialist training or that their interest lies in that direction. The overseas-qualified are more likely to mention the first reason and the British-qualified the second. (This difference arises because more of the overseas-qualified do, in fact, have specialist training to a high level). It is significant that 16 per cent of overseas-qualified GPs who would prefer a hospital career said in explanation that this would be their preference if they could get a senior post in the chosen specialty, whereas none of the British-qualified gave this explanation (Table A41). Other reasons given for preferring a hospital career are (i) that hospital work is more varied and interesting; (ii) that dealing with serious illnesses is more interesting, or (iii) dealing with trivial complaints and sorting out patients' personal problems ('social medicine') is boring.

The main reasons given for preferring to remain in general practice relate to freedom and independence and to the type of work. Basing percentages on GPs who wish to remain GPs, we found that as many as 42 per cent of the British-qualified and 31 per cent of the overseas-qualified mentioned the greater independence of the GP, and a further 15 per cent and 12 per cent of the two groups respectively mentioned the rigid, bureaucratic, authoritarian or impersonal nature of hospitals (Table A42). Under the heading of the type of work, involvement with people or the opportunity to 'treat people, not illnesses' is seen as an advantage of general practice by 41 per cent of the British-qualified and 38 per cent of the overseas-qualified. The more varied work of a GP and the continuity of involvement with patients and families was also often mentioned.

The general conclusion to be drawn from these findings is that most GPs are fully reconciled to a career in general practice, if they did not choose it in the first place, and in support of their position they can argue that general practice offers strong positive advantages over a specialist career. However, a proportion of late entrants still feel that their career is a second best, or that they are out of place in general practice, and because there are far more late entrants among the overseas-qualified, there are also substantially more who see themselves as misfits than among the British-qualified. The point can be further underlined by one further finding. A significant proportion of overseas-qualified GPs (18 per cent) had already obtained membership or fellowship before they went into general practice. Among this group as many as 61 per cent still say that they would prefer to be hospital doctors.

Characteristics of a general practice

The NHS has adopted a policy of encouraging group practices on the ground that they are able to provide a more comprehensive service. Overseas-qualified doctors tend to be concentrated in the smaller and particularly in the single-doctor practices that are now being discour-

Table VII.3 Number of doctors in the practice by type of area (Q96)

Column percentages

Size of practice	Total (British and overseas quali-fied)	British-qualified			Overseas-qualified		
		Total	Conurb-ation	Other	Total	Conurb-ation	Other
1	11	10	13	8	22	28	18
2	15	13	13	13	32	32	33
3	23	23	15	26	17	15	18
4	21	22	22	22	14	14	15
5-6	23	25	23	25	10	9	11
7 or more	6	7	11	5	2	2	2
Not stated	1	1	3	—	2	1	3
Mean practice size	3.66	3.81	3.94	3.76	2.68	2.50	2.81
Base: All GPs							
Unweighted	*730*	*477*	*137*	*340*	*253*	*110*	*143*
Weighted	*1,923*	*1,549*	*425*	*1,224*	*274*	*124*	*150*

NB: Since this table is based on individuals and not on practices, it shows the distribution of practice sizes and mean practice size of the practices to which a sample of individuals belong. This is different from the distribution of practice sizes and mean practice size as such (the latter would be substantially smaller than shown). The analysis is by the country of qualification of the individual sampled; the practice as a whole may contain a mix of British and overseas-qualified doctors.

aged. We found that 22 per cent of overseas-qualified GPs, compared with 10 per cent of the British-qualified, belong to single-doctor practices. Further, as many as 54 per cent of overseas-qualified GPs belong to one or two-doctors practices, compared with 23 per cent of the British-qualified. The mean practice sizes for the two groups of doctors are 2.68 and 3.66 respectively.[1] As was pointed out in Chapter II, overseas-qualified GPs tend to be concentrated within the conurbations, but this does not seem to explain their concentration in small practices. When the comparison was confined to GPs within conurbation areas, it was found that the overseas-qualified belong to smaller practices than the British-qualified (the means are 2.50 and 3.94 respectively). The reason why overseas-qualified GPs tend to be in small practices is not known from the survey. It is possible that they find it more difficult than the British-qualified to gain positions in group practices, for which there may be more demand.

---

1 That is, the mean practice size of the practices to which a sample of individual doctors belong: see the note to Table VII.3.

An analysis by length of service as a GP shows that doctors with longer service are markedly more likely to belong to the smaller, and specifically to the single-doctor, practices. Of course, this emphasises the difference between doctors qualified in Britain and overseas in this respect. The overseas-qualified tend to have much shorter service than the British-qualified, yet in spite of this they tend to belong to small practices. If we consider only GPs who have been in general practice in Britain for up to five years, we find that among the British-qualified the mean size of practice is 4.4 doctors, compared with 2.9 among the overseas-qualified (Table A43).

Some indication of the amount of work to be done by the doctors in a practice is given by the number of patients on the list in relation to the number of doctors. Of course, this is a very crude indicator, since the incidence of illness will vary according to local conditions and the demographic and socio-economic characteristics of the people on the list. Informants were asked how many patients there were on the list for the practice as a whole, and this figure was then divided by the number of doctors. Unfortunately, because of a technical error, the exact number of patients was not coded where this was more than 10,000 (which it was in 31 per cent of the practices to which our sample of GPs belonged). In the practices for which we have exact information, we found that the median number of patients per doctors was 2,090 (Table VII.4), and there was no significant difference between the practices to which British and overseas-qualified doctors belong. It is interesting to find a wide variation among all groups in the number of patients per doctor. For 21

Table VII.4   Number of patients per doctor

Column percentages

	Total	British-qualified	Overseas-qualified
1- 750	8	9	5
751-1500	13	14	10
1501-1875	19	19	17
1876-2250	23	22	30
2251-3000	28	28	28
3001 or more	9	9	9
Median number of patients	2,090	2,060	2,180
Base: Doctors in practices with less than 10,000 patients *Weighted*	*1,324*	*1,098*	*223*

NB The table shows the total number of patients on the list of the practice divided by the number of doctors (including any assistants or trainees). Practices with 10,000 or more patients (to which 31 per cent of the sample of GPs belong) are not included because of a technical error.

per cent of the practices covered, the figure is up to 1,500 whereas for 9 per cent it is over 3,000.

Informants were also asked to estimate what proportion of the practice's patients were 'coloured'. Although these figures were estimates rather than exact counts, the overall mean of 4.36 per cent is reasonably close to the actual proportion of the population who are coloured (which is about 3.5 per cent) which suggests that the estimates were fairly realistic ones. Overseas-qualified doctors tend to have a substantially higher proportion of coloured patients on their lists than British-qualified doctors (the mean percentages are 7.74 and 3.76 respectively). This directly follows from the geographical distribution of overseas-qualified GPs that has already been mentioned. Nevertheless it is rare for more than 30 per cent of an overseas-qualified GP's patients to be coloured.

Table VII.5 Percentage of patients in the practices who are coloured

Column percentages

Per cent of coloured patients	Total	British-qualified	Overseas-qualified
		Informant is:	
None	29 ⎤ 65	30 ⎤ 67	23 ⎤ 52
One	36 ⎦	37 ⎦	29 ⎦
2-3	9	9	12
4-5	8	8	4
6-9	2	2	3
10-15	7 ⎤	6 ⎤	9 ⎤
16-29	3 ⎥ 15	2 ⎥ 12	5 ⎥ 27
30 or more	5 ⎦	4 ⎦	13 ⎦
Mean	4.36	3.76	7.74
Base: All GPs			
Unweighted	*730*	*477*	*253*
Weighted	*1,923*	*1,649*	*274*

More central to our interest is the ethnic mix of doctors in the same practice. If country of qualification were irrelevant to doctors applying for a place in a practice and to those selecting from among applicants, then we would expect to find that British and overseas-qualified doctors would have the same chance of having an overseas-qualified doctor in the practice (other than themselves). Because of the different geographical distribution of the two groups, we would admittedly expect the actual situation to depart from this model slightly. In fact, there is a fairly marked tendency for doctors belonging to minority groups to be clustered within the same practices. Excluding single-doctor practices, which in this context are irrelevant, we found that 15 per cent of British-qualified GPs belong to practices in which there is a 'coloured' doctor, whereas 57 per cent of overseas-qualified GPs belong to practices in which there is a 'coloured' doctor other than the informant. The more detailed findings show that there is little tendency for doctors belonging to a particular ethnic group (for example, Indians) to be in a practice containing other doctors belonging to that particular group. Rather, there is a general tendency for coloured doctors, regardless of the particular ethnic group, to cluster together. There is no tendency for doctors from white anglophone countries to be grouped with other (coloured) overseas-qualified doctors.

Table VII.6   Ethnic mix of doctors in the same practice (Q.99)

Column percentages

	Total	Informant qualified in:		
		UK/Eire	Else-where	Indian sub-continent[1]
Practice includes one or more doctors belonging to the following groups, apart from the informant:				
White British	91	96	55	52
White anglophone	8	8	7	8
Other white	4	3	7	7
Any white	**94**	**98**	**64**	**61**
Indian	13	9	44	48
Pakistani or Bangladeshi	4	3	9	11
Other Asian	3	3	5	5
Other coloured or black	1	1	4	4
Any Asian	**19**	**14**	**54**	**60**
Any coloured or black	**20**	**15**	**57**	**63**
Base: GPs in practices of two or more doctors				
Unweighted	*607*	*417*	*190*	*155*
Weighted	*1,686*	*1,479*	*207*	*166*

1 Informants in this column are also included in the previous one.

Although the tendency for coloured doctors to group together is quite strong, many practices still contain a mixture of white and coloured doctors. Thus, 55 per cent of the practices to which an overseas-qualified doctor belongs also contain one or more white British doctors (Table VII.6), and, as already mentioned, 15 per cent of practices to which a British-qualified doctor belongs also contain a coloured doctor. This tendency towards ethnic grouping may arise because doctors tend to seek positions in practices containing other doctors belonging to their own group, or because of differential (and possibly discriminatory) selection criteria on the part of British or overseas-qualified doctors, or from a combination of all three factors.

Pattern of working

The hardest information that we have about the amount of work done by GPs comes from a series of questions on the number of home visits made, the number of patients seen at the surgery, and the number of weekends and weekday nights spent on call. In addition, GPs were asked how many hours they had worked in one full week[1], but the answers to this question can be regarded as reflecting an attitude rather than giving a reliable estimate of something definable. Since GP's hours of work are not fixed, and since they are themselves responsible for organising their working pattern as they see fit, what constitutes work as opposed to leisure is bound to be open to widely different interpretations.

The findings suggest that consultations at the surgery outnumber home visits by about five to one. While overseas-qualified GPs tend to see more patients at the surgery than those British-qualified, they tend to make fewer home visits. The average figures for surgery consultations are 179 per week for the British-qualified and 223 per week for the overseas-qualified, while the averages for home visits are about 37 per week for the British-qualified compared with about 29 for the overseas-qualified. The total volume of work undertaken by the two groups would be the same on the assumption that one home visit takes about the same amount of time as five surgery consultations. Thus the two groups seem to handle about the same amount of work.

The difference in the balance between surgery consultations and home visits among the two groups seems to imply a difference in the style of practice. Doctors in the conurbations tend to make fewer visits to patients, but, if anything, to see more patients in surgery, as might be expected from the fact that their practices are less dispersed. However, these differences between type of area are not nearly enough to explain the differences between British and overseas-qualified GPs. For example, if we consider only GPs in conurbations, we still find that among the overseas-qualified there is a greater emphasis than among the British-qualified on surgery consultations as opposed to visits (Table VII.7).

There are also different styles of practice as between the different generations among British doctors as Table A44 shows. Older British doctors make substantially more home visits than younger ones, which probably means that over time GPs are tending to see more of their patients at the surgery rather than at home.

The questions about the number of weekends and weekday nights during which the GP is on call can also be expected to produce reasonably reliable information. The findings show that, on average, GPs are on call

---

1 That is, the last full week prior to the one during which the interview was carried out.

Table VII.7   Mean number of visits to patients and surgery consultations, by type of area (Qs 104 and 105)

	Mean number per week:	
	Visits to patients	Surgery consultations
All GPs	36.1	185
British-qualified		
Total	37.4	179
of which:		
Conurbation	33.9	181
Other areas	38.7	178
Overseas-qualified		
Total	28.5	223
of which:		
Conurbation	24.7	232
Other areas	31.8	215

during 1.2 weekends out of every four (Table VII.8 and Tables A45 and A46), and during 6.1 weekday nights out of every twenty. In each case, overseas-qualified GPs are substantially more often on call than British-qualified. To a large extent, this is because they tend to belong to smaller practices, particularly to single-doctor ones, in which doctors tend to be more often on call because few or no alternates are available. When the number of doctors in the practice is controlled, there is still some tendency for the overseas-qualified to be more often on call than the British qualified, but the difference is slight. The pattern of on-call arrangements is little related to whether or not the practice is in a conurbation area.

GPs claimed that they worked an average (mean) of 63 hours in the week before the questionnaire was completed, but this mean figure conceals a considerable amount of variation. Ten per cent of GPs said they had worked for up to 35 hours and 20 per cent 86 hours or more. This wide variation partly reflects unevenness in hours worked from one week to the next (bearing in mind that the question referred to a specific week). In fact, 36 per cent of GPs said that the previous week's hours were unusually short or long (18 per cent that they were unusually short and exactly the same proportion that they were unusually long). However, further analysis emphasises that this is only a partial explanation. For example, even among those who said that the previous week's hours were shorter or the same as usual, 13 per cent claimed to have worked for 86 hours or more; and even among those who said that the previous week's

Table VII.8   Weekends and nights on call (Qs 106-109).

Column percentages

	Total	British-qualified	Overseas-qualified
Number of weekends on call out of every four			
Never on call at weekends	10	10	11
Less than one	19	20	7
One	43	45	32
Two	21	20	27
Three	1	*	3
Four	6	4	18
Not stated	1	1	1
Mean	1.21	1.12	1.75
Number of weekday nights on call out of every twenty			
Never on call weekday nights	9	8	11
One-two	5	5	6
Three-four	33	35	20
Five-six	19	21	10
Seven-eight	12	11	15
Nine-ten	8	8	10
Eleven-nineteen	7	6	13
Twenty	5	4	12
Not stated	3	3	3
Mean	6.1	5.8	8.0
Base: All GPs			
Unweighted	*730*	*477*	*253*
Weighted	*1,923*	*1,649*	*274*

hours were longer or the same as usual, 8 per cent claimed to have worked for 35 hours or less. From these wide variations, it seems likely that different GPs interpret the idea of 'work' in different ways.

The major activities of GPs about which we have information are surgery consultations and visits to patients. It is useful to consider how the information about activities can be reconciled with the estimates of working hours. It might be assumed, for example, that of the average 63 hours work in a week, 10 hours was spent on activities other than seeing patients (for example, reading medical literature, attending courses or discussion groups, discussing cases with colleagues, administration of the practice). Of the remaining 53 hours, 15 might be spent in making 30 visits to patients, on the assumption that each visit takes about half an hour including travelling time. This would leave 38 hours for consultations at the surgery, or 7½ hours of surgeries on each of five days, during which an average of 170 patients would be seen, or roughly one every

Table VII.9 **Hours worked during one week (Q.102)**

Column percentages

	Total	British- qualified	Overseas- qualified
Up to 25	4	4	4
26-35	6	6	6
36-45	16	17	11
46-55	21	22	14
56-65	16	16	15
66-85	17	17	19
86-105	9	9	11
106 or more	11	10	18
Not stated	1	1	2
Mean	63.0	61.8	69.5
Base: All GPs			
Unweighted	*730*	*477*	*253*
Weighted	*1,923*	*1,649*	*274*

thirteen minutes. This is one way in which the two sets of information (about activities and working hours) could be reconciled, although it may alternatively be thought that the major activities are performed in a shorter time than is assumed here, and that a higher proportion of claimed working hours is spent on activities other than the major ones of surgery consultations and visiting patients. A much more detailed study of GPs' working patterns would have to be carried out in order to understand the matter fully.

While we cannot place too much reliance on the absolute number of hours per week that GPs claim to work it is perhaps significant that overseas-qualified GPs claim to work longer hours (mean 69.5) than those qualified in Britain (61.8). This is not because the two groups tend to handle different volumes of work, for we have already seen that the volumes of work handled by each group is about the same. GPs in single-doctor practices tend to claim longer hours than others, and this has some bearing on the longer hours of overseas-qualifed GPs, but some difference remains when the size of the practice is controlled. It might be suggested that the differences between the two groups in terms of age and years of experience in general practice are relevant in this context, but analysis by length of GP experience does not help to explain the difference in hours worked. The findings seem to show that overseas-qualified GPs either actually take longer to handle the same volume of work as British GPs, or think they do (Tables A47 and A48).

Answers to the questions on the use of deputising services to attend to

GPs' calls shows that these services are now extensively used in the conurbation areas, but much less extensively elsewhere. In the conurbation areas, 80 per cent of GPs sometimes use deputising services, and among these are 67 per cent who use them regularly during one or more types of period: 39 per cent during holiday periods, 47 per cent during normal weekends and again 47 per cent during normal weekdays (presumably at night). Outside the conurbations, only 25 per cent of GPs ever use deputising services.

Table VII.10   Use of deputising services, by type of area (Qs 110-111)

Column percentages

	Total	Conurbation areas	Other areas
Never used	59	19	75
Ever used	41	80	25
Regularly used for:			
Holiday periods	23	39	16
Normal weekends	27	47	19
Normal weekdays	26	47	18
Sometimes used, but not at any of these periods	5	13	1
Not stated	*	1	*
Base: All GPs			
Unweighted	*730*	*247*	*483*
Weighted	*1,923*	*549*	*1,374*

Overseas qualified GPs are nearly twice as likely to use deputising services as the British-qualified, but this is probably entirely because their practices tend to be in areas where the services are available. There is no difference in the proportion using the services as between British and overseas-qualified doctors within the conurbations; the majority of doctors in the conurbations make use of the services regardless of their country of qualification. Among GPs outside the conurbations, the overseas-qualified are about twice as likely to use the services as the British-qualified, but this is probably because of a different geographical distribution of the two groups across the non-conurbation areas. Outside the conurbations, the overseas-qualified GPs may tend to have practices in urban settings where the services are available, while the British-qualifed may be more likely to have practices in rural or suburban settings where there are no deputising services for them to use.

In single-doctor practices, the use of deputising services may be a necessity, but in larger practices it should be easier for doctors to arrange a rota that gives them continuous cover. It is therefore surprising to find (Table A49) that the use of deputising services is not very consistently

e

related to the size of practice, and that the services are extensively used even among large group practices: 37 per cent of doctors in practices of six or more use the services, most of them on a regular basis.

Table VII.11   Use of deputising services, by British and overseas-qualified and type of area (Qs 110-111)

Column percentages

	Total	British-qualified			Overseas-qualified		
		Total	Conur-bation	Other	Total	Conur-bation	Other
Never used	59	62	12	77	36	15	53
Ever used	41	37	78	22	64	84	47
Regularly used for:							
Holiday periods	23	31	38	14	34	40	30
Normal weekends	27	24	45	16	46	54	39
Normal weekdays	26	25	50	16	36	38	34
Sometimes used, but not regularly at any of these periods	5	4	14	1	6	12	1
Not stated	*	1	1	*	*	1	—
Base: All GPs							
Unweighted	*730*	*477*	*137*	*340*	*253*	*110*	*143*
Weighted	*1,923*	*1,649*	*425*	*1,224*	*274*	*124*	*150*

We found that 40 per cent of GPs do some hospital work in addition to their work in general practice. Among this 40 per cent, the mean number of sessions worked at the hospital is 2.3 per week. There are no significant differences here between British-qualified GPs and those who qualified overseas. Hospital work is one additional item that could in practice have been counted towards hours worked in the week previous to the survey (although interviewers were instructed, when a query arose, to advise informants to exclude it). However, over GPs as a whole, hospital work amounts to only 0.8 of a session, on average, per week, and would therefore make a difference of only two or three hours in the time worked. This does not materially affect the preceding discussion.

Relationships with colleagues and patients
The great majority of GPs in group practices think they have excellent (60 per cent) or good (29 per cent) relationships with their partners. There is no significant difference between British and overseas-qualified doctors in this respect. Relationships with partners are not significantly affected by the ethnic composition of the practice; relationships are generally thought to be good whether or not the other partners belong to the same ethnic group as the informant.

In the last chapter we showed that there was more awareness of language difficulties in communicating with other doctors and with patients among British-qualified than among overseas-qualified hospital doctors. Both groups of doctors ascribed any difficulties to the inadequacy of other people's English rather than to the inadequacy of their own[1]. The findings for GPs are very similar, except that the difficulties of communication are rather less emphasised by both groups of GPs, probably because the language competence of overseas-qualified GPs is, in fact, substantially higher than that of overseas-qualified hospital doctors, who have generally spent a much shorter time in the UK.

Among GPs, 43 per cent of British-qualified compared with only 6 per cent of those qualified elsewhere think that they sometimes have language difficulties in communicating with other doctors. These difficulties are generally thought to be moderate (17 per cent of the British-qualified), or slight (21 per cent), but rarely severe (4 per cent). Just under half of British-qualified GPs (49 per cent) compared with 20 per cent of the overseas-qualified are aware of language difficulties in communicating with patients. The difficulties of which both groups are aware lie in communicating with members of ethnic minority groups: only 2 per cent of overseas-qualified GPs admit to difficulties in communicating with white English-speaking patients. In support of this, our objective test of command of English (see Chapter III) does show that the standard of English of most overseas-qualified GPs is high.

We found among hospital doctors that British-qualified doctors were twice as likely as those qualified elsewhere to think that some English patients dislike being treated by a coloured doctor and to consider that this led to problems. The findings of GPs are again similar. Seventy-two per cent of British-qualified think there is some patient resistance of this kind, compared with only 31 per cent of those qualified elsewhere. More than half of the British-qualified (51 per cent) think this is a serious or slight problem, compared with 15 per cent of the overseas-qualified. These questions are, of course, attitudinal rather than factual. The findings show that many British-qualified GPs are critical of the ability of overseas-qualified doctors to communicate in English to other doctors and patients, and that many believe that the overseas-qualified also have other problems in their relationships with patients caused by a degree of reserve or prejudice on the part of the patients; overseas doctors tend not to be aware of such difficulties. This contrast of attitudes and perceptions can be summed up by saying that British doctors are inclined to be critical of overseas doctors, while overseas doctors are inclined not to be self-critical.

Future plans

The great majority of overseas-qualified GPs have now settled permanently in the UK; only 11 per cent expect to leave in the foreseeable

1 See pages 95-97

future, among whom are 6 per cent who expect to return to the country of origin (the balance of 5 per cent intend to move on to another country). The proportion of British-qualified GPs who intend to leave the country in future is very small indeed (3 per cent). The vast majority of GPs, whether British or overseas-qualified, intend to remain in general practice (97 per cent of the British-qualified and 94 per cent of the overseas-qualified).

VIII   Attitudes Towards Asian Doctors and Selection Procedures

There are two important questions which lie behind much of the discussion of the findings of this study, but which the study is not able to confront directly. The first of these is whether the level of medical competence is generally as high among overseas doctors as among British doctors, or whether it is high enough, bearing in mind the jobs which these doctors have to perform. The information about command of English, qualifications and experience which has already been presented has some relevance to the general level of competence, but the light which it casts on the question is an uncertain one. It was not possible to go further than this with the methods available.

The second important question is how far overseas-qualified doctors are fairly treated by selection and promotion procedures. Here, the analysis of career progress in relation to qualifications and experience in Chapter V is relevant, but we have no direct measure of the fairness of selection and promotion procedures themselves. It is, therefore, a matter for discussion how far the relatively slow progress of some overseas-qualified doctors is a consequence of unfairness in the system, or how far of other factors; it could still be argued that the explanation lies in variables which the study was not able to measure adequately.

As to the facts, and the correct analysis of the facts, we cannot take the discussion on these two questions any further, although a few indications will emerge from the findings of more qualitative research at nine hospitals to be presented in the next chapter. However, we do have substantial findings on the attitudes and views of doctors (both British and overseas-qualified) on these questions, and these findings are important in defining the climate of opinion within which any policy initiatives would be taken. A series of detailed questions was included at the end of the interview to establish whether doctors *believe* that the level of competence of Asian doctors is lower than that of white British doctors, and whether they believe that an appreciable proportion of Asian doctors are below a minimum acceptable standard. A further series of questions explores doctors' *views* about the fairness of selection procedures, and to this can be added some factual information about the numbers of applications made by British and overseas-qualified doctors before finding a suitable job. These questions are not, and they are not intended to be, objective measures of the actual level of competence of Asian doctors, or of the fairness of selection procedures. They are, however, a useful measure of the climate of opinion among doctors on these issues.

Attitudes towards Asian doctors

Towards the end of the interview, informants were directly asked to compare the level of competence of white British and Asian doctors. The questions were asked about Asian doctors (rather than about overseas-qualified doctors as a whole) because informants are likely to perceive Asians as a group and to be ready to make generalisations about them, where they might be reluctant to generalise about all overseas doctors. At the same time, Asians are much the largest group among overseas doctors; they account for two-thirds of the overseas-qualified.

There were two groups of questions, each of which was worded in a scrupulously neutral way (to an extent that made them sound somewhat pedantic). In the first group, informants were asked whether on average the competence of Asian and white British doctors was similar or different, and if different, which group of doctors had the higher level of competence on average. The limitation of these questions is that they take no account of the possible range of variation in competence among the two groups of doctors. To take account of this, we risked a second, rather complex, group of questions in which doctors were asked to say whether the variation of competence was greater among Asians or among white British doctors or about the same among the two groups. Where informants said that there was more variation among one or the other group, they were asked whether that group contained a higher proportion of outstandingly good doctors and (separately) whether it contained a higher proportion of doctors below a minimum acceptable standard. It would, of course, be perfectly consistent for the informant to answer 'yes' to both of these questions.

The first thing to be said about the findings is that the great majority of doctors (whether British-qualified or not) are prepared to play this game. Only 16 per cent of doctors qualified in the UK and 15 per cent of those qualified elsewhere failed to give a definite answer to the first group of questions, and for the second group, these figures were rather lower. These findings suggest that country of qualification or ethnic group (or more probably a mixture of the two) is generally regarded as an indicator of competence and as an important factor informing the judgements that doctors make of their colleagues. Doctors may be generalising on the basis of their personal experience; in that case, for a group having extensive scientific training, they seem prepared to make rather sweeping generalisations. On the other hand, doctors may have formed their judgement of the overseas-qualified from statements made in the Merrison report, which concluded that 'there are substantial numbers of overseas doctors whose skill and the care they offer fall below that generally acceptable in this country'. They may also have interpreted the withdrawal of recognition for the purposes of full registration from Indian medical colleges in 1975 as implying dissatisfaction on the part of the GMC about the standard of training at these colleges. It may, therefore, be factors such as these which have influenced individual doctors, rather than their personal experience; this would certainly help to explain the considerable unanimity of opinion which, as we shall see, these questions reveal.

Similar proportions of doctors are ready to say:

(i) that British doctors are, on average, more competent than Asians, and

(ii) that there is more variation of competence among Asian doctors, among whom there is a higher proportion who are below a minimum acceptable standard.

The group of doctors who agree to each of these propositions is probably virtually the same. Their view is that the general level of competence is lower among Asians, that there is among Asians a relatively high proportion of doctors who are below a minimum acceptable standard, that there is greater variation of competence among Asians, but there is not, among Asians a relatively high proportion who are outstandingly good doctors.

Table VIII.1 Perceived level of competence of Asian and British doctors, by country of qualification

Column percentages

	Country of qualification:					
	UK/ Eire	White anglo-phone country	Indian sub-con-tinent	Arab country	Else-where	Overseas less white anglo-phone
British are more competent than Asians	60	43	16	40	42	22
Asians are more competent than British	*	1	3	3	2	3
Level of competence is similar	23	25	69	44	32	61
Don't know	16	30	12	13	25	14
Base: All informants						
Unweighted	*1,016*	*73*	*664*	*111*	*117*	*892*
Weighted	*3,382*	*104*	*748*	*119*	*137*	*1,004*

Q164 I would like you to compare the level of competence of Asian and white British doctors in the National Health Service. First would you say that *on average* the competence of Asian and white British doctors is similar or different?
Q165 If different, which of the two groups do you think has the higher level of competence on average?

From the first group of questions, we found that 60 per cent of British-qualified doctors believed that the average level of competence is lower among Asian than among white British doctors (Table VIII.1). This compares with 43 per cent of doctors qualified in white anglophone countries, 41 per cent of those qualified in other countries overseas apart from the Indian sub-continent, and 16 per cent of those qualified in the Indian sub-continent (who are essentially the 'Asians' mentioned in the question). Less than 0.5 per cent of British-qualified doctors, and also negligible proportions of the other groups (including Asians) say that the average level of competence of Asian doctors is higher than that of white British doctors.

From the second group of questions, we found that 59 per cent of British-qualified doctors thought that the variation of competence is greater among Asian than among white British doctors, and 51 per cent thought that there is, among Asians, a higher proportion who are below a minimum acceptable standard (Table VIII.2). It would have been open to these informants to maintain, at the same time, that there is also, among Asians, a higher proportion who are outstandingly good doctors, but only two per cent of British-qualified informants took this view. The responses of the various groups of overseas-qualified doctors stand in the same relation to those of British-qualified doctors here as at the first group of questions.

An important feature of these findings is that overseas-qualified doctors, other than Asians, have a marked tendency to be critical of Asian doctors. For example, 40 per cent of those qualified in an Arab country think that the average level of competence of Asian doctors is lower than that of white British doctors. A majority of Asian doctors take the view that the standards of the two groups are similar: 69 per cent say that the average level of competence is similar, and 59 per cent that the variation in competence is about the same. However, where Asian doctors did think there was a difference between the standards of the two groups, their answers were generally critical of their own group. For example, 16 per cent said that the average level of competence of Asian doctors is lower than that of white British doctors, while only 3 per cent took the opposite view. Thus, while there is a contrast between the views of British and Asian doctors, these views are not diametrically opposed.

These responses amount to a forthright expression, among British doctors, of the view that the level of competence is comparatively low among Asian doctors, with a less forthright expression of the same view among overseas doctors other than Asians, and with the Asians themselves dissenting, but less strongly than they might. An external point of reference will help to show how forthrightly British doctors express these views compared with other groups in a comparable situation. In 1974, PEP carried out a survey of a national sample of employers at plant level in order to explore policies and practices in relation to racial

Table VIII.2   Perceived variation in competence among Asian and British doctors, by country of qualification (Qs 166-170)

	UK/ Eire	White anglo-phone country	Indian sub-con-tinent	Arab country	Else-where	Overseas less white anglo-phone
Variation of competence is:						
Greater among Asians	59	55	28	40	32	30
Greater among white British	2	1	2	6	7	3
About the same	28	29	59	42	42	55
Don't know	10	14	10	13	20	12
Variation is greater among Asians:						
A higher proportion of Asians are out-standingly good	2	1	5	2	3	5
A higher proportion of Asians are below minimum acceptable standard	51	36	14	29	22	17
Variation is greater among white British:						
A higher proportion of British are out-standingly good	2	1	1	3	3	1
A higher proportion of British are below a minimum acceptable standard	*	—	1	1	—	1
Base: All informants						
Unweighted	*1,016*	*73*	*664*	*111*	*117*	*892*
Weighted	*3,382*	*104*	*748*	*119*	*137*	*1,004*

discrimination and disadvantage.[1] At a late point in the interview, employers were asked a series of questions which invited them to compare British, West Indian, Indian and Pakistani workers in various respects. One series of questions covered manual workers, and a separate series non-manual workers. About one-half of employers refused to make generalisations about the comparative qualities of manual workers belonging to the various ethnic groups, and about 70 per cent refused to

[1] See David J. Smith, *Racial Disadvantage in Employment*, PEP No. 544 (June 1974)

make such generalisations as far as non-manual workers were concerned. Compared with employers, doctors are much readier to make generalisations about the competence of those belonging to a particular ethnic group, and the generalisations that they make are much more strongly critical. For a profession that is trained to take a cautious and analytic approach, this amounts to a very forthright expression of views.

Further analysis shows that there is little relationship between doctors' views on this issue and the amount and nature of contact with Asian doctors that they are likely to have had. The views of hospital doctors and GPs are almost identical, although hospital doctors will generally have substantially more experience of working with Asian doctors. Young doctors have the same views as older doctors, and the views of men and women are similar, although men are, if anything, slightly more critical of Asian doctors. Analysis by grade of post among British-qualified hospital doctors shows that while those at all grades are strongly critical of Asians, consultants are markedly more critical than those at lower grades; thus, 81 per cent of British-qualified consultants said that the average level of competence of Asian doctors was lower than that of white British doctors. Among overseas-qualified doctors, too, consultants are rather more likely to be critical of Asians (39 per cent of consultants compared with 23 per cent of those at lower grades subscribe to the same proposition). This difference by grade of post could well result from a difference in the nature of experience (specifically, consultants will often have had supervisory responsibility for Asian doctors). However, on the other side of the question, even the youngest and most junior doctors are strongly critical of Asians, so that the main body of these attitudes is not demonstrably related to doctors' personal experience.

We emphasised at the beginning of this chapter that these findings relate to doctors' views and not to the actual facts of the situation. Whether or not the facts accord with these views, it seems likely that the views have had, and will have, an effect on appointments committees. If the level of competence among Asian doctors is not, in fact, significantly lower than among British doctors, then Asian applicants will tend to be consistently under-rated. If the level of competence among Asians does, in fact, tend to be lower, then individual Asian applicants of a high standard will tend to be under-rated through being classified as members of a group whose standards tend to be low. As we have already stressed, we have no direct evidence about the fairness of selection procedures, and it is possible that selection committees set all generalisations about Asian doctors on one side when considering applications. All that we can say is that doctors make such generalisations so readily that to set them aside would require a considerable conscious effort.

Although hospital doctors and GPs as a whole hold much the same views as to the relative competence of Asian and British doctors, some additional findings do emerge when more detailed analyses are carried out within each of these groups. In the case of GPs, we found no significant difference between the views of white British doctors who have and do not have colleagues in the practice belonging to an ethnic minority group. This confirms the point that these views are fairly independent of the amount and nature of contact with Asian doctors. In the case of hospital doctors, we found some tendency among the British-qualified for those in the youngest age group (up to 29) to be less critical of Asians; for example, 50 per cent of those in this age group, compared with 78 per cent of older British-qualified hospital doctors believe that the average level of competence of Asians is lower than that of white British doctors.

Views on the fairness of selection procedures

All informants were asked a series of questions to establish their views of selection procedures for medical hospital jobs. The questions were addressed to GPs as well as hospital doctors because all British GPs and nearly all overseas-qualified GPs have themselves had hospital jobs in Britain at some time. The questions set up a hypothetical situation in which two doctors applied for the same job, one coloured and overseas-qualified and the other white and British-qualified. It was stated that these two hypothetical applicants had 'comparable qualifications and experience', but what was regarded as 'comparable' in this context was not further defined. Informants were asked whether, in their opinion, these two applicants would have the same or different chances of being offered the job. Those who thought that the coloured and overseas-qualified applicant would be rejected more often than the white British applicant were asked to say in their own words what made them think so, and were subsequently asked which of a series of interpretations of the behaviour of selection boards they agreed with.

The questions were framed in this way after a pilot enquiry had shown that many doctors believed that a coloured and overseas-qualified applicant would generally be at a disadvantage, but believed at the same time that selection boards had good or at any rate understandable reasons for behaving in this way. So that informants should have the opportunity to express this kind of view, we did not specify that the two hypothetical applicants were identical in every way except for the colour of their skin, but instead allowed the informant to put his own interpretation on 'comparable qualifications and experience'. This meant that informants were able to answer on the assumption that what was formally comparable was not comparable in fact, but they were also able to say that unfair discrimination occurred if that was their view.

The great majority of informants (86 per cent) said that the coloured and overseas-qualified applicant would be rejected more often than the white and British-qualified applicant in the situation described; exactly half of informants thought he would be rejected much more often, while 36 per cent thought he would be rejected slightly more often. Virtually no informants (less than 0.5 per cent) thought that the coloured and overseas-qualified applicant would tend to be favoured, only 6 per cent thought the two applicants would have equal chances, while the remaining 8 per cent refused to express an opinion. As in the case of the questions on the competence of Asian doctors, this amounts to a most forthright expression of views on a matter of which the majority of informants can have no direct experience. It is again striking that such a small proportion refuse to answer.

Table VIII.3 Perception of overseas doctors' chances when applying for hospital jobs, by type of job and British and overseas qualified

Column percentages

	Total	GPs	Hospital doctors	British-qualified	Overseas-qualified
Equal chances	6	7	6	6	8
White British applicant rejected:					
Slightly more often	*	*	*	*	*
Much more often	*	*	*	*	*
Coloured overseas-qualified applicant rejected:					
Slightly more often	36	36	36	38	29
Much more often	50	46	52	48	56
Don't know	8	11	5	8	7
Base: All informants					
Unweighted	*1,981*	*730*	*1,251*	*1,016*	*965*
Weighted	*4,490*	*1,923*	*2,567*	*3,382*	*1,108*

Q171 Suppose that two doctors with comparable qualifications and experience, one of them coloured and overseas-qualified, the other white and British-qualified, apply for the same hospital job in England. In this situation, what do you think will be the chances of the two applicants? Please choose a statement from this card. (The card showed fuller versions of the statements shown in the table.)

British-qualified and overseas-qualified doctors are substantially in agreement on this issue. The same proportion of the two groups believe that the coloured and overseas-qualified applicant will tend to be disfavoured, but the overseas-qualified are rather more likely to think that he will be rejected much more often as opposed to slightly more often (56 per cent compared with 48 per cent). There is little difference between the views of hospital doctors and GPs, and what little difference there is reflects the lesser experience of GPs; thus, 11 per cent of GPs compared with 5 per cent of hospital doctors refused to answer.

What these findings show is that the great majority of doctors, whether British or overseas-qualified, believe that coloured and overseas-qualified applicants are at a disadvantage when applying for hospital jobs. They do not show that the great majority believe that selection boards unfairly discriminate. The further questions, however, allow us to define these views more closely. The first, open, question was phrased as follows: 'What makes you think that the coloured overseas applicant will tend to be rejected more often?'. The kind of answer that this question strictly expects is one which mentions evidence available to the informant about the behaviour of selection committees or the chances of different sorts of applicant. However, another kind of answer that is frequently given is about the reasons that selection boards have for rejecting coloured overseas-qualified applicants. Our classification of answers takes separate account of these two kinds of response. First, every informant was assigned to one of a number of mutually exclusive groups according to the kind of evidence that he provided to support the view that selection committees tend to reject coloured and overseas-qualified applicants. Secondly and separately, the reasons given for the selection boards' behaviour were classified in a scheme which allowed the same informant to give a number of different reasons. It should be noted that in Tables VIII.4-5, which present the findings, percentages are based on all informants (including those who do not believe that overseas-

Table VIII.4   Evidence of preference for a British-qualified applicant (Q.172)

Column percentages

	Total	UK/Eire	White anglo-phone country	Elsewhere
			First qualified in:	
Total who think overseas applicant would be disfavoured	86	86	83	86
Type of evidence:				
Personal experience as an applicant	6	4	2	12
Personal experience as a member of selection committees	2	3	3	*
Experience of friends/from observing who is appointed to jobs	6	6	7	6
Assertion that it is generally assumed/thought/known that British qualifications are preferred, but no specific evidence mentioned	50	49	59	52
No evidence mentioned	21	24	13	15
Base: All informants				
Unweighted	*1,981*	*1,016*	*73*	*892*
Weighted	*4,490*	*3,382*	*104*	*1,004*

129

Table VIII.5   Reasons for preferring British-qualified applicants for hospital jobs (Q172)

	Total	First qualified in:		
		UK/Eire	White anglo-phone country	Elsewhere
Competence or likely competence				
Inadequate English of overseas-qualified/(slight) language difficulties	19	22	21	6
Overseas qualifications are of uncertain value, British qualifications are known and understood	13	16	9	5
Overseas qualifications or training tend to be of lower value	10	11	25	5
Overseas-qualified doctors tend to be/are reputed to be less competent	5	6	10	2
British doctor can perform better since he knows the culture	5	6	4	1
Overseas doctors hard to assess, some good, some bad	3	4	2	1
Communication/knowledge of culture especially important in psychiatry	2	2	—	*
Overseas/Asian doctors are less responsible or reliable	1	1	1	*
Overseas doctors are aggressive/ have a different attitude to patients	1	1	2	—
Overseas doctors are too respectful or passive	*	*	—	*
Overseas doctors put lower value on human life/have different attitudes to pain	*	1	—	—
Any mention of competence	43	51	51	18
Prejudice or preference				
Prejudice/colour prejudice/ chauvinism	14	15	29	9
Consultants prefer to work with people from their own background/whose assumptions they share	10	11	11	5
British doctors are preferred for senior posts	1	1	1	1
Prejudice against women combined with prejudice against overseas doctors	*	*	—	*
Any mention of prejudice or preference	23	26	39	14

Table VIII.5 (cont'd)

| | Total | First qualified in: | | |
		UK/Eire	White anglo-phone country	Elsewhere
The preference is explicable				
Natural/inevitable to prefer your own people/kind	23	17	10	44
British doctors should be preferred since they will stay permanently	3	3	2	3
Any mention that preference is explicable	25	20	11	46
Relationship with colleagues and patients				
Patients prefer white/British doctors, the employer must take account of this	5	6	4	1
Problems of integration/difficult relationships between white and British doctors	3	4	4	*
Any mention of relationships	7	9	7	2
Others				
British doctors get better references	1	2	—	1
Other reasons for the preference	1	1	1	2
No reasons mentioned	11	9	15	18
British-qualified applicant would not be preferred/don't know	14	14	17	14
Base: All informants				
Unweighted	*1,981*	*1,016*	*73*	*892*
Weighted	*4,490*	*3,382*	*104*	*1,004*

qualified applicants are disfavoured) so that the proportion of all informants holding a particular view can immediately be seen.

A majority of informants (71 per cent) can either provide no evidence to support a view that coloured and overseas-qualified applicants are rejected or simply state that it is generally known or assumed that this is the case. Twelve per cent of overseas-qualified doctors excluding white anglophones, and 6 per cent of the total, say that they have knowledge from personal experience as an applicant, while 3 per cent of the British-qualified and of white anglophones say they have knowledge from personal experience as a member of selection committees (less than 0.5 per cent of doctors qualified elsewhere claim this kind of experience). Finally, 6 per cent of doctors, with no variation by country of qualification, say they have knowledge from the experience of friends or

131

from observing who is appointed to jobs. The main thrust of these findings is that the generally forthright views of doctors that coloured and overseas-qualified applicants tend to be rejected are based on hearsay or on what is generally assumed to be the case rather than on hard evidence (which would, for most doctors, be hard to come by). However, 12 per cent of overseas-qualified doctors (excluding white anglophones) think they have personal experience of treatment by a selection board which they presumably consider to be unfair.

The reasons given to explain the more frequent rejection of coloured overseas-qualified applicants are mostly attempts to 'justify' the behaviour of selection committees or at least to make it understandable. Most informants (whether British or overseas-qualified) do not believe that the more frequent rejection of overseas-qualified applicants with 'comparable qualifications and experience' amounts to an unfair or discriminatory practice. Those who mention prejudice, colour prejudice or chauvinism are a group who definitely do believe that the practice is unfair or discriminatory. These amount to 14 per cent of the total, and account for 15 per cent of the British-qualified, 29 per cent of white anglophones, but only 9 per cent of other overseas-qualified doctors. Thus overseas-qualified doctors (other than white anglophones) are *less* likely to make allegations of unfair or discriminatory practices than British-qualified doctors. It is interesting that white anglophones are substantially more likely than other groups to make allegations of this kind. This is probably because they are in a more detached and neutral position, as they are not involved, either as victims or as agents, in the practices in question.

An important proportion of informants (10 per cent) say that consultants prefer to work with people from their own background, whose assumptions they share, who will laugh at their jokes, and so on. These informants do not make it clear whether they think that this preference is a reasonable one, so we cannot say whether they regard the result as unfair or discriminatory . Altogether 23 per cent of informants say that British-qualified applicants are favoured either because of a prejudice or because of a preference more neutrally expressed. Again, far more white anglophones (39 per cent) than other overseas doctors (14 per cent) give one of these kinds of answer; the British-qualified are more likely than the overseas-qualified to answer in this kind of way (26 per cent compared with 14 per cent).

All other answers appear to be attempts to explain or justify the rejection of overseas applicants. The answers most frequently given by British-qualified and white anglophone doctors were ones that cast doubt on the competence or likely competence of the overseas-qualified applicant. In fact, 51 per cent of the British-qualified, and exactly the same proportion of white anglophones, gave answers of this kind, compared with only 18 per cent of other overseas-qualified doctors. The answers most frequently given by overseas-qualified doctors other than white anglophones are ones which seek to justify rejection of coloured and overseas-qualified applicants on the ground that it is natural or inevitable to prefer your own people or your own kind. Just under half of the overseas-qualified doctors apart from white anglophones gave answers of this kind, compared with only 11 per cent of white anglophones and 20 per cent of British-qualified doctors.

The answers characteristically given by British-qualified doctors and white anglophones, which cast doubt on the competence or likely competence of the coloured, overseas-qualified applicant, can be taken in two different ways. On the one hand, they may amount to a rejection of the premise that the qualifications and experience of any two applicants are comparable, given that one is coloured and overseas-qualified and the other white and British. On this interpretation, informants are saying that the overseas applicant will be rejected because he is, as an individual, inferior to the white British applicant according to criteria which are properly and justifiably applied. Alternatively, these informants may be saying that coloured and overseas-qualified applicants as a group tend to have less competence in various ways than white British applicants, and that a selection committee is justified in rejecting an overseas applicant because he belongs to a group which is generally less competent, although they do not know whether, as an individual, he is more or less competent than the white British applicant with whom he is competing. Some of the answers in particular can be taken in this way, for example, the assertion that overseas qualifications are of *uncertain* value, or that overseas doctors *tend* to be less competent. In fact, of course, inferior treatment of an individual because of his membership of a group whose general characteristics he may or may not share is discriminatory under the law. To the extent that informants are seeking to explain the behaviour in these terms, they are interpreting it as behaviour that is, in fact, discriminatory, although they do not themselves consider it in that light.

The answer characteristically given by overseas doctors (other than white anglophones) is that it is natural to prefer your own kind. This appears to amount to an admission that the practice is unfair and discriminatory, while providing a weak justification for it on the basis that unfairness and discrimination is 'only human nature'.

A final group of answers relates to relationships with colleagues and patients. Nine per cent of British-qualified doctors justify rejection of coloured overseas-qualified applicants on the ground that patients prefer white British doctors, or refer to difficulties in relationships between white British and coloured overseas doctors. A similar proportion of white anglophones (7 per cent) but a very small proportion of other overseas doctors (2 per cent) gave this kind of answer.

A second follow-up question was added in order to obtain a clearer and more definite indication of how informants interpret the alleged behaviour of selection committees in tending to reject coloured overseas-qualified applicants. In this question, three possible attitudes on the part of selection boards were directly put to informants: (i) that they put a lower value on overseas qualifications, (ii) that they believe that the overseas doctor is less likely to be competent to practise in Britain, and (iii) that they (the selection committees) discriminate against coloured overseas-qualified doctors on racial or ethnic grounds. In addition, the first two attitudes were presented in two alternative forms: for example, 'they rightly put a lower value on overseas qualifications', 'they wrongly put a lower value on overseas qualifications'. It was open to the informant to agree with two or with all three of the basic attitudes, but not, of course, to say that the same attitude on the part of selection committees was both right and wrong.

Table VIII.6 shows that 38 per cent of informants think selection boards tend to reject coloured overseas-qualified applicants because they put a lower value on overseas qualifications, 46 per cent because they believe that 'the overseas doctor is less likely to be competent to practise in Britain' and 18 per cent because the selection boards discriminate

Table VIII.6 Reasons for selection boards rejecting coloured overseas-qualified applicants (Q173)

Column percentages

	Total	First qualified in:		
		UK/Eire	White anglo-phone country	Elsewhere
They put a lower value on overseas qualifications				
— rightly	29	35	23	8
— wrongly	9	5	10	22
— rightly or wrongly	38	40	33	30
They believe that the overseas doctor is less likely to be competent				
— rightly	33	41	31	6
— wrongly	12	7	17	30
— rightly or wrongly	46	48	48	36
They discriminate on racial or ethnic grounds	18	18	28	18
Don't know	16	15	11	20
Not relevant[1]	14	14	17	14
Base: All informants				
Unweighted	*1,981*	*1,016*	*73*	*892*
Weighted	*4,490*	*3,382*	*104*	*1,004*

[1] Informants who did not say that the coloured, overseas-qualified applicant would be disfavoured.

against coloured overseas-qualified doctors on racial or ethnic grounds. On this basis (that is, without considering whether the attitudes of the selection boards are considered to be 'justified' or not) there is substantial agreement between British and overseas-qualified doctors in the interpretations given. British-qualified doctors are somewhat more likely than those qualified elsewhere (other than white anglophones) to think that a lower value is put on overseas qualifications (40 per cent compared with 30 per cent) and that overseas doctors are thought likely to be less competent (48 per cent compared with 36 per cent), but the level of agreement between the two groups is more striking than the contrast. Exactly the same proportion of the two groups subscribe to the view that selection boards discriminate on racial or ethnic grounds (18 per cent), but this compares with a significantly higher proportion of white anglophones (28 per cent). Thus, those who might be involved in discrimination as actors or as victims hold the same views about its incidence, while a neutral group, which does not identify itself with either party, is significantly more likely to think that discrimination occurs. This can be understood on the assumption that British doctors prefer to believe that discrimination does not occur because they identify themselves with the group which would then be responsible for an unfair practice, and coloured overseas doctors also prefer to believe the same thing because they do not want to feel that their own group is openly under attack. In the case of white anglophones, however, allegations of discrimination do not diminish their self-respect in either of these ways, and can therefore be made more freely.

Although there is substantial agreement between British-qualified doctors and those who qualified elsewhere on the reasons that selection boards have for their alleged rejection of coloured and overseas-qualified applicants, there is sharp disagreement as to whether the reasoning of selection boards is correct or not. For example, 41 per cent of British-qualified doctors say that selection boards *rightly* believe that the overseas doctor is less likely to be competent to practice in Britain, compared with only 6 per cent of overseas-qualified doctors (excluding white anglophones). The pattern of answers here is rather complex, because informants might agree with more than one interpretation of the selection boards' behaviour. To overcome this difficulty, the summary table, Table VIII.7 sorts informants into three basic groups: (i) those who gave only approving answers (that the selection boards would rightly make one or other of the judgements about the overseas applicant; (ii) those giving only disapproving answers (that the selection boards would wrongly make one or other of the judgements, or that they would discriminate on racial or ethnic grounds); and (iii) those giving mixed answers (both an approving and a disapproving answer). When informants who could not say why selection boards would tend to favour the white British applicant, and those who did not believe that they would, are included in the table, it adds up to 100 per cent.

Table VIII.7   Why selection boards reject coloured overseas-qualified applicants in summary, by country of qualification (Q173)

Column percentages

	Total	UK/Eire	White anglophone country	Elsewhere
		First qualified in:		
Only approving answers	37	46	22	9
Only disapproving answers	22	13	33	53
Mixed answers	11	12	17	4
Don't know	16	15	11	20
Not relevant	14	14	17	14
Base: All informants				
Unweighted	*1,981*	*1,016*	*73*	*892*
Weighted	*4,490*	*3,382*	*104*	*1,004*

The summary table shows that there is a very strong contrast between British and overseas-qualified doctors in their evaluation of the behaviour of selection boards. Nearly half of British-qualified doctors (46 per cent) think that selection boards disfavour overseas applicants and approve of their reasons for doing so, compared with only 9 per cent of overseas-qualified doctors (excluding white anglophones). Only 13 per cent of the British-qualified doctors wholly disapprove of the selection boards' alleged behaviour, compared with 53 per cent of the overseas-qualified. The responses of white anglophones are midway between these extremes.

Further analysis of these views of selection procedures for hospital jobs is best confined to hospital doctors, since (unlike GPs) they are personally involved. Analysis by grade of post together with country of qualification shows that each of these factors is separately related to the view that overseas-qualified doctors are rejected for good reasons. Those who are consultants and those who are British-qualified are likely to hold this view, and consequently, British-qualified consultants hold it most strongly of all (56 per cent gave wholly approving answers), and overseas-qualified junior doctors least strongly of all (9 per cent). Conversely, the view that overseas-qualified doctors are rejected for poor reasons or because of discrimination is held least strongly by British-qualified consultants, although here there is little, if any, difference among overseas-qualified doctors between consultants and juniors. Thus, as many as 40 per cent of overseas-qualified consultants, (compared with 42 per cent of overseas-qualified junior doctors) gave answers wholly disapproving of selection boards. It is important to notice, therefore, that concern about bias or discrimination is strong among overseas-qualified doctors at all levels. Among British-qualified doctors, the juniors quite often share this concern, but consultants very seldom do.

Table VIII.8   Why selection boards reject coloured overseas-qualified applicants in summary: hospital doctors by grade and country of qualification

	British-qualified:		Overseas-qualified:	
	Consultants	Other grades	Consultants	Other grades
Only approving answers	56	32	20	9
Only disapproving answers	5	21	40	42
Mixed answers	12	18	10	4
Don't know	14	22	22	21
Not relevant	13	7	8	24
Base: Hospital doctors				
Unweighted	*201*	*318*	*85*	*603*
Weighted	*786*	*886*	*101*	*805*

Column percentages (above table)

Analysis of overseas-born hospital doctors by year of coming to the UK (Table VIII.9) shows that the earliest migrants (those who came up to 1959) are a special group whose views are similar to those of British doctors; in fact, many of them are British-qualified, and comparatively few of them are Asians. Among migrants who came from 1960 onwards, there is only a slight tendency for earlier migrants to give answers that are more approving of selection boards. It is more important to stress that even among overseas doctors who have been in the UK for fifteen years,

Table VIII.9   Why selection boards reject overseas-qualified applicants in summary: hospital doctors born abroad by year of coming to the UK (Q173)

	Year of coming to the UK:			
	Up to 1959	1960-1964	1965-72	1973-1978
Only approving answers	43	20	11	7
Only disapproving answers	16	41	52	51
Mixed answers	11	19	3	5
Don't know	21	14	21	24
Not relevant	9	6	13	13
Base: Hospital doctors born abroad				
Unweighted	*109*	*50*	*209*	*441*
Weighted	*146*	*70*	*253*	*505*

Column percentages (above table)

137

about half believe that selection boards are biassed or that they discriminate against overseas qualified doctors. This is a view that many overseas doctors retain after many years of experience.

Personal experience of discrimination
When asked what makes them think that a coloured overseas-qualified applicant for a hospital job will tend to be rejected, we have seen that 12 per cent of overseas-qualified doctors (less white anglophones) mention their personal experience as an applicant. However, many informants when answering this question are concerned to elucidate the attitudes and behaviour of selection boards rather than to explain what kinds of evidence they have for thinking that a coloured overseas-qualified applicant will tend to be disfavoured. Thus the figure of 12 per cent gives an indication of the proportion of overseas doctors who will spontaneously mention personal experience of discrimination in answer to a more general question about the chances of different kinds of applicant. In addition, coloured doctors (who account for 86 per cent of the overseas-qualified) were asked directly 'Do you believe that you have yourself been rejected when applying for a hospital post because of ethnic or racial discrimination?'. Just over one-fifth (22 per cent) answered 'yes'. From further questions about 'the occasion when the evidence was most clear cut' we find that most of those doctors who claim personal experience of discrimination cannot provide clinching evidence that discrimination actually occurred. Only 5 per cent were told that another applicant was preferred because he was white and British; 33 per cent found that the white British doctor appointed was a weaker candidate than themselves, 8 per cent felt that it was clear from the interview that there was prejudice against them, and the remainder were basing their allegation on weaker evidence than this.

The 'occasion on which the evidence was most clear cut' was within the past year in 24 per cent of cases, between two and five years ago in 39 per cent of cases, and more than five years ago in 33 per cent of cases (for the remaining 4 per cent there was no information on this point). These findings eliminate the possibility that claims of personal experience of discrimination relate to practices that have recently died out. In the majority of cases the job applied for was at senior house officer (37 per cent) or registrar level (33 per cent), but it is interesting that in 13 per cent of cases the informant was applying for a consultant post.

Even this question about personal experience of discrimination is attitudinal rather than factual. The findings tell us little about informants' actual experiences, but they do tell us something important about how they interpret these experiences. It is rare in any social context for a coloured person to be told that he is being rejected because he is coloured. It follows that even where discrimination is widespread it is rare for the victims to have clear evidence that it has occurred in a particular case. They would have to gain access to a much larger body of

Table VIII.10   Reasons for thinking that rejection was based on discrimination (Q.178)

	Per cent
I was told that a white British (qualified) applicant would be preferred	5
The white British doctor appointed was a weaker candidate than I	33
It was clear from the interview that there was (racial) prejudice against me	8
The white British (qualified) doctor appointed had no better qualifications than I	4
I was not offered an interview although I had the required qualifications and experience	5
I was not appointed although I had the required qualifications and experience	24
The candidate appointed was also coloured/overseas-qualified, so on second thoughts there was no discrimination	1
No evidence/can't prove it/maybe I was wrong to think there was discrimination	3
Other answers	9
Don't know/not stated	7

Base: Coloured doctors who claim to have been rejected for a hospital job because of discrimination
Unweighted	*205*
Weighted	*240*

NB Where the informant mentioned more than one reason, only the highest in the above list was counted.

facts about the field of applicants than is normally available to them. Even where the facts are available, the statement that discrimination occurred is an interpretation of the facts in the light of certain criteria, and there is room for different people to choose different criteria or to apply them differently. For example, some might regard it as justifiable to treat basic medical qualifications obtained outside Britain as inferior to British ones, while others might regard this as a weak justification of what is essentially racial or ethnic discrimination. It is not even clear what is the correct interpretation of the law on this point until the matter is tested in the courts, and it has not yet been tested.

Therefore, what informants are being asked is whether they have had an experience as an applicant which they choose to interpret as one of discrimination. It is not in the least surprising that most of those who answer 'yes' can cite no very specific evidence that discrimination actually occurred, and this does not imply in the slightest that their allegations are unjustified, but merely reinforces the point that applicants are not, in the nature of the case, in a position to have clinching evidence. Equally, of course, from the fact that one-fifth of coloured doctors claim experience of discrimination, it does not in the least follow that in these cases discrimination actually occurred. We do not have objective evidence about the fairness of selection procedures against which to test these allegations.

However, to help us to evaluate the findings it is worth referring to another study in which such objective evidence was also obtained.[2] As part of a study of racial disadvantage carried out between 1973 and 1976, PEP interviewed a nationally representative sample of people of Asian and West Indian origin, and as part of this survey, informants were asked whether they believed that employers discriminated against coloured applicants and whether they had personal experience of discrimination as an applicant. Considering only the findings for men, we found that about one-half of Asians and about three-quarters of West Indians believed that employers discriminate, while 14 per cent of Asians and 16 per cent of West Indians thought they had had personal experience of discrimination as applicants. At the same time, it was established from a series of rigorously controlled field experiments that an Asian or West Indian applicant for an unskilled or semi-skilled manual job would face discrimination in 46 per cent of cases, for a skilled manual job in at least 22 per cent of cases, and for a white-collar job in at least 30 per cent of cases. Since a single person has usually made many job applications, it follows that a majority of Asians and West Indians have, in fact, been victims of discrimination in this context at some time, whereas only about 15 per cent believe that they have.

In the present case we find that the great majority of doctors (whether belonging to racial minority groups or not) believe that coloured overseas-qualified applicants will tend to be disfavoured, but a comparatively small proportion (about one-fifth) are prepared to say that this is because of discrimination. In the more general survey, alternative explanations of a tendency to reject coloured applicants were unlikely to apply, particularly to that majority of the population who were manual workers. Thus, the rejection of coloured applicants was generally equated by informants with discrimination. This is the most striking difference between the two sets of findings. Coloured overseas-qualified doctors, unlike Asians or West Indians generally, are likely to look for other interpretations of the rejection of their group instead of discrimination. The proportion claiming personal experience of discrimination is comparable in the two cases, but if anything higher among coloured doctors than among Asians and West Indians generally. In the case of the general study, these rather modest claims of personal experience of discrimination are accompanied by much more substantial and widespread actual discrimination than the claims would suggest. Whether or not the same applies in the case of doctors, we do not know.

---

2 David J. Smith, Racial Disadvantage in Britain, Penguin Books, 1977

But if discrimination on the part of hospital selection committees were substantial and widespread, we would still expect to find claims of personal experience of discrimination at the level actually encountered.

The proportion claiming personal experience of discrimination, which is best regarded as an indication of the level of feelings of grievance, does vary substantially between different groups of coloured doctors. It is, if anything, higher among those who are now GPs than among those who are now hospital doctors (27 per cent compared with 20 per cent), which fits in with other indications that overseas doctors have in some cases become GPs because of failure to progress in the hospital service. Older and more senior hospital doctors, and those who have been in the UK for longer are substantially more likely to claim personal experience of discrimination than younger or more junior hospital doctors or those who recently arrived in the UK. This suggests that doctors tend to conclude that they have been subject to discrimination after long experience, rather than hastily. It does not seem to imply that discriminatory acts (as perceived by coloured doctors) have diminished in recent years, since we have already seen that many of the experiences of discrimination cited occurred in recent years (in 63 per cent of cases the 'occasion on which the evidence was most clear cut' was within the past five years).

Doctors with a good command of English are substantially more likely than those whose English is poor to claim experience of discrimination.

Table VIII.11 Claims of personal experience of discrimination when applying for hospital jobs: coloured doctors by various factors

	Per cent claiming personal experience
All coloured doctors	22
Present job	
General practitioner	27
Hospital doctor	20
Hospital doctors by grade:	
House Officer/Senior House Officer	14
Registrar	19
Senior Registrar	42[1]
Medical Assistant/Consultant	37
All coloured doctors by country of qualification:	
UK/Eire	16
Indian sub-continent	23
Arab country/Iran	19
Elsewhere	27

141

Table VIII.11 (cont'd)

	GPs	Per cent claiming personal experience Hospital doctors
Age:		
Up to 29 years	n.a.	10
30-34 years	17[1]	15
35-44 years	32	28
45 years and over	22	40
Sex		
Male	29	22
Female	19	11
Qualification		
Membership or Fellowship	45	32
No Membership or Fellowship	23	16
Coloured doctors born abroad by year of coming to the UK		
Up to 1959	15	44
1960-64	33	41
1965-69	31	33
1970-72	33[1]	24
1973-74	n.a.	14
1975-76	n.a.	12
1977-78	n.a.	4
Coloured doctors by language test score:		
0-14	n.a.	12
15-18	32[1]	19
19-23	35	19
24-25	26	20
26-27	27	30
28-29	30[1]	52[1]

[1] Low base (unweighted less than 30)

Q.175 Do you believe that you have been rejected when applying for a hospital job because of ethnic or racial discrimination?

It could be argued from this that doctors whose English is poor tend to discount experiences of rejection because they know they have a definite handicap. However, all the other evidence about command of English suggests that doctors with poor English tend to be unaware of their handicap. It is probably that the longer experience of older doctors and those who have been in this country for longer is the prime factor; those who have had long experience are more likely to have come to the conclusion that they have been subject to discrimination and are also more likely to speak English well. However, the relationship with command of English does at least suggest that claims of discrimination do not mostly relate to rejections which were actually the result of the applicant's inadequate English. Men are substantially more likely than women to claim that they have experienced ethnic or racial discrimination, possibly because women are equally or more concerned about sex discrimination.

Number of job applications made

In order to gain an indication of how far overseas-qualified doctors are rejected when applying for hospital jobs, informants were asked how many applications they had made before finding their present job, and also in how many cases they were offered an interview. Because it would be rare for a person to go on making applications after having received the offer of a job and for two job offers to be made simultaneously, the total number of applications made is a good indicator of the chances that any particular application has of being finally accepted. The further information on the number of invitations to an interview shows whether rejections tended to occur before or after the interview stage.

If we had found that overseas-qualified doctors made no more applications before finding a job than British-qualified doctors, this would be good, though not conclusive, evidence that discrimination did not occur (not conclusive because overseas doctors might tend to apply for more junior or less desirable jobs than similarly qualified British doctors). To the extent that there is a tendency for overseas-qualified doctors to have made more job applications, this leaves room for the possibility that discrimination has occurred, although the findings merely set an upper limit to possible discrimination, since a higher incidence of rejection of the overseas-qualified could be for justifiable reasons.

In fact there is a large difference between the number of job applications made by the two groups. The majority of British-qualified hospital doctors (76 per cent) made one, two or three job applications, and only 8 per cent made seven or more Among the overseas-qualified doctors (excluding white anglophones) there is also a substantial group of doctors who made one, two or three applications (43 per cent). Thus, among both groups there is a large proportion of doctors who had no serious difficulty in finding the present job. However, among the overseas-qualified there is also a substantial minority who made large numbers of applications: 22 per cent made 7-25 applications, and 17 per cent made 26 or more, and among this latter group is an appreciable number of doctors who made very large numbers of applications indeed — for example, 6 per cent made 99 or more White anglophones made about the same number of applications as British-qualified doctors.

There are two kinds of contrast here between British and overseas-qualified doctors. First, there is among the overseas-qualified a much greater variation in the numbers of applications made: a substantial proportion made many. Secondly, the overseas-qualified made, on average,

Table VIII.12 Number of job applications made before finding present job: hospital doctors by country of qualification (Q. 187)

Column percentages

| | First qualified in: | | |
	UK/Eire	White anglophone country	Elsewhere
One	48	40	31
2-3	28	39	12
4-6	12	13	11
7-25	6 ⎤ 8	5 ⎤ 5	22 ⎤ 39
26 or more	2 ⎦	— ⎦	17 ⎦
Job obtained without making a formal application	2	2	4
Not stated	1	1	2
Mean number of applications	3.1	2.6	16.5
Base: All hospital doctors			
Unweighted	*539*	*60*	*652*
Weighted	*1,733*	*84*	*749*

NB The full distribution, which is summarised in this table, shows that some overseas-qualified doctors made very large numbers of applications; this accounts for the high mean.

many more applications than the British-qualified. The mean number of applications made is 16.5 for the overseas-qualified (excluding white anglophones) compared with 3.1 for the British-qualified, a ratio of more than five to one. More details are shown in Table VIII.12.

If we are thinking of the proportion of doctors who encountered difficulties in finding the present job, then these means should not be considered. In that context, the important finding is that 39 per cent of the overseas-qualified (excluding white anglophones) compared with 8 per cent of the British-qualified made seven or more applications. The overseas-qualified doctors who encountered serious difficulties, while a substantial group, are still a minority. However, if we are thinking of the responses made by selection committees to applications received, the means are relevant, because they give an indication of the number of applications from doctors belonging to the two groups that are rejected. An application from a British-qualified doctor has a one in three chance of being accepted, whereas one from an overseas-qualified doctor has only a one in sixteen chance.

This last statement is an over-simplification, of course, because there are substantial numbers of overseas-qualified doctors for whom the chances of acceptance are similar to those of British-qualified doctors, while there are also substantial numbers who are rejected many times by different selection committees. These different committees appear to apply similar criteria which lead to the rejection of the same group of overseas doctors. It seems that these criteria are applied mainly on the basis of the initial application and without the benefit of references, since the doctors who make many applications also tend to have been offered few interviews. If, for example, we consider the group of doctors who made at least ten applications for each interview they were offered, we find they account for 37 per cent of overseas-qualified doctors (excluding white anglophones) compared with only 4 per cent of British-qualified doctors. Thus, the bulk of the rejections of these doctors who make many applications occur at the shortlisting stage and not after an interview.

One possible explanation of the difficulties of some overseas-qualified doctors is that they find it hard to become established when they first arrive in the UK. Selection committees might have a strong tendency to turn down applications from doctors who have as yet had no experience of British medicine. Analysis by year of coming to the UK does show that those who arrived more recently find it more difficult to get a job, but it seems to make little difference whether the doctor arrived five years ago or within the past year. Doctors who have been in the UK for many years are substantially less likely to encounter great difficulties, but even among those who came between 1964 and 1969, 34 per cent had to make seven or more applications to find their present job. Thus, the exceptional difficulties of some overseas-qualified doctors do not only relate to the first job or even to the second, but to several subsequent ones as well.

There is a strong tendency, among the overseas-qualified, for those at the lower hospital grades to have made more applications than those at the senior grades, and something of the same tendency is apparent among British-qualified doctors except that consultants do not fit in with the trend. This, combined with the fact the overseas doctors are concentrated within the more junior grades, accounts for some of the contrast between the two groups, but it is not a very important factor. Thus, the contrast in the number of applications made remains when the comparison is made within each particular grade, except that there is no difference in the case of consultants. If, for example, we consider only senior house officers, we find that among the overseas-qualified 52 per cent made seven or more applications, compared with 7 per cent of the British-qualified.

Overseas-qualified doctors whose English is poor had to make substantially more applications than those whose English is good, and this may be a prime factor that partly accounts for the greater difficulties of the newly-arrived and more junior. Also, imperfect English may account for a substantial component, but by no means all, of the higher incidence of rejection of the overseas-qualified compared with the British-qualified. If we confine our attention to hospital doctors whose English is perfect (those who score 28-29 on the test) we find that among

145

the British-qualified only 6 per cent made seven or more applications, compared with 22 per cent of the overseas-qualified, and the mean numbers of applications made by the two groups were 2.8 and 8.8 respectively.

These findings strongly confirm the opinion held by the great majority of doctors that overseas-qualified applicants (most of whom are coloured) are more likely to be rejected than white British applicants when applying for hospital jobs. However, it seems that this is true of a particular group of overseas doctors rather than overseas doctors as a whole. Those at junior grades, who have arrived recently and whose English is poor are rather likely to fall into the group which has difficulties; nevertheless, some senior overseas doctors, who have been in the UK for some years and whose English is perfect, have also had exceptional difficulties. There must, therefore, be other criteria applied by selection boards on the basis of written applications only according to which a subset of overseas doctors is being continually rejected.

These findings set a high upper limit to the amount of discrimination that may occur. While accepting them, it can still be argued that discrimination does not occur at all, but only on the assumption that a substantial minority of overseas-qualified applicants are less well-qualified or less competent than the British-qualified applicants with whom they compete for the same jobs.

Although our findings on views of the selection process for hospital jobs are complex in detail, they can be briefly summarised in outline. British and overseas-qualified doctors are agreed that a coloured overseas-qualified applicant is likely to be rejected when in competition with a white British applicant having similar qualifications and experience. British doctors generally think that the rejection of the overseas-qualified applicant is explicable either on the ground that overseas qualifications are inferior or on the ground that overseas-qualified doctors are likely to be less competent to practise in the UK. Overseas-qualified doctors agree that rejections occur because qualifications are thought to be inferior or because overseas applicants are thought to be less competent to practise in the UK, but they believe that these judgements are misguided. Only about one-fifth of doctors, whether British or overseas-qualified, believe that there is discrimination on racial or ethnic grounds against coloured overseas-qualified applicants for hospital jobs, and only one-fifth of coloured and overseas-qualified doctors think that they have themselves been subject to such discrimination. The view, held by most doctors, that coloured overseas-qualified applicants tend to be rejected when in competition with white British applicants, is strongly confirmed by information about actual rejection rates. How far this is actually the result of discrimination remains an open question.

The selection procedure for jobs in general practice

Doctors were asked a series of questions which broadly parallel those relating to the hospital service, about the selection procedure for general practice; some modifications to the questions were introduced to fit the different circumstances. Views about the chances of coloured overseas-qualified applicants were again sought by setting up a hypothetical situation in which two doctors with comparable qualifications and experience applied for the same job, one of them white and British, the other coloured and overseas-qualified. However, in the case of general practice, it was necessary to ask the question twice, once for the case where the other doctors in the practice were coloured and overseas-qualified, and again for the case where they were white and British-qualified. In this way, we were able to establish whether informants thought that coloured and overseas-qualified GPs would tend to disfavour white British applicants as well as whether they thought that white British GPs would tend to disfavour coloured and overseas-qualified applicants. This complication did not arise in the case of hospital jobs because selection committees are nearly always dominated by a white British point of view even if they sometimes contain one or more overseas-qualified consultants. Where informants said that one or other type of applicant would tend to be disfavoured, they were simply asked whether this was because of ethnic or racial discrimination or for some other reason. (In the case of hospital jobs they were asked a more detailed question about which of a number of possible factors, including discrimination, was involved.)

Both hospital doctors and GPs were asked these questions. The views of hospital doctors are very similar to those of GPs, except that a larger proportion of hospital doctors could express no definite opinion, presumably through lack of experience. The analysis presented here will be confined to GPs, who are more likely to have informed opinions on this subject.

We shall first consider the hypothetical case where a practice consisting entirely of coloured and overseas-qualified doctors is looking for another partner. Among British-qualified GPs, only 10 per cent thought that a coloured overseas-qualified applicant and a white British applicant would have equal chances in this situation. A majority (61 per cent) thought there would be a tendency for a white British applicant to be disfavoured, and a significant minority (8 per cent) thought that he would tend to be favoured; 21 per cent had no definite opinion. Among overseas-qualified GPs, a substantially higher proportion thought that the two applicants would be given equal chances (32 per cent, compared with 10 per cent of the British-qualified). About half of the overseas-qualified thought that one or other applicant would tend to be disfavoured; (24 per cent thought that the white British applicant would tend to be disfavoured and 24 per cent thought that it would be the overseas qualified applicant). The remaining 20 per cent had no definite opinion. A substantial minority of British-qualified GPs (36 per cent) thought that there would be a tendency towards unequal treatment because of racial or ethnic discrimination, compared with a smaller minority of overseas-qualified GPs (16 per cent).

Table VIII.13   Opinions on the chances of rejection of coloured overseas-qualified and white British applicants for jobs in general practice: British and overseas-qualified GPs (Qs. 179-182)

Column percentages

	Where practice consists of coloured overseas-qualified doctors		Where practice consists of white British doctors	
	British-qualified informant	Overseas-qualified informant	British-qualified informant	Overseas qualified informant
Equal treatment	10	32	7	17
White British applicant rejected:				
Slightly more often	29	17	*	2
Much more often	32	7	—	*
Coloured overseas-qualified applicant rejected:				
Slightly more often	5	12	33	27
Much more often	3	12	52	39
Don't know	21	20	8	15
Unequal treatment due to discrimination	36	16	38	27
Base: GPs				
Unweighted	*477*	*253*	*477*	*253*
Weighted	*1,649*	*274*	*1,649*	*274*

These findings show that there is sharp disagreement between British and overseas-qualified GPs about the preferences of overseas-qualified doctors who are looking for a partner. The proportion who thought that there would tend to be some preference for one or the other group is markedly different, but more striking than this, a much higher proportion of the British-qualified thought that the white British applicant would tend to be disfavoured. It is interesting that a significant proportion of British and of overseas-qualified GPs believed that overseas-qualified doctors would prefer to be joined in the practice by a white British doctor, but a much higher proportion of the overseas-qualified than of the British-qualified held this view.

These findings clearly show that informants do not believe that a tendency to favour white British or coloured overseas-qualified applicants is confined to the majority group. Where it is the minority group which is doing the selection there are two possible motives for a preference. One is a desire to work with others belonging to the same ethnic group, or in other words, ethnic solidarity. The other is a desire to raise the prestige of the practice by including in it doctors belonging to the majority group, or perhaps to broaden the range of social and cultural skills possessed by the practice as a whole. British doctors give much the greatest weight to ethnic solidarity, although some of them think the second motive is important. Overseas-qualified doctors give equal weight to a desire to integrate with the majority group. On the assumption that a preference for British-qualified doctors can more easily be justified on the grounds of their superior qualifications, training or suitability for general practice in the UK, it follows that overseas-qualified GPs are less likely to think that racial or ethnic discrimination occurs, for the preference that they have in mind is more often a preference for a white British doctor that might be justified in these terms.

We now turn to the case where a practice consisting entirely of white and British-qualified doctors is looking for another partner. Here there is a measure of agreement between British and overseas-qualified GPs that the coloured overseas-qualified applicant will tend to be rejected more often (85 per cent of the British-qualified compared with 66 per cent of the overseas-qualified). Negligible proportions of either group believe that the white British applicant will tend to be rejected more often, and fairly similar proportions of the two groups think that actual discrimination will be involved (38 per cent of the British-qualified, 27 per cent of the overseas-qualified). Thus there is fairly widespread agreement that a coloured overseas-qualified applicant will be at a disadvantage, and a substantial minority of GPs think that this is because of ethnic or racial discrimination.

If the findings for the two situations are taken together, British-qualified doctors are more likely than those qualified elsewhere to think that the selections made by GPs will tend to reflect an ethnic preference or one based on country of qualification, and they are also more likely to think that discrimination occurs. Both groups of doctors are more likely to think that white British doctors will show an ethnic preference when considering applicants than to think that coloured overseas-qualified doctors will do so.

In general terms, there is a fairly broad consensus of opinion among GPs that preferences as between white British and coloured overseas-qualified doctors enter into the selection process for jobs in general practice, and a substantial minority of GPs believe that racial or ethnic discrimination enters into this. There is rather more emphasis on discrimination in this context than in the case of selection for hospital jobs. This could be because the form of the questions was slightly different, but it may well be that doctors think discrimination is more likely to occur where, as in the case of general practice, the selection process is more informal and involves a smaller number of people.

Doctors who had ever applied for a job in general practice (42 per cent of the total) were asked 'Do you believe that you have yourself been rejected when applying for a job in a general practice because of ethnic or racial discrimination?'. Among the relevant overseas-qualified doctors, 15 per cent said they had experienced discrimination. This is similar to the proportion of coloured doctors who believe they have faced discrimination when applying for hospital jobs (20 per cent). In the case of applications for jobs in general practice, white British doctors who had made such applications were also asked whether they thought they had ever faced discrimination: only 2 per cent answered 'yes'.

Overseas-qualified GPs made, on average, twice as many applications as British-qualified GPs before finding their present job (9.1 compared with 4.4). Although this contrast is a sharp one, it is less marked than in the case of hospital doctors (15.0 applications on average for overseas-qualified hospital doctors compared with 3.1 for the British-qualified). However, in the case of hospital doctors, some of the overall difference is accounted for by differences in the grade of post applied for and in the language competence of the two groups. In the case of GPs there are no different grades of post to consider (medical assistants and trainees were not included in the sample), and differences in language competence between British and overseas-qualified GPs have little relevance. The number of applications made by overseas-qualified GPs does not vary consistently according to language test score, and if we confine our attention to those with perfect English (scoring 28-29 on the test) we find that the overseas-qualified still made, on average, 9.6 applications compared with 4.0 for the British-qualified, a ratio of more than two to one. While this contrast is not as strong as the overall contrast shown in the case of hospital doctors, it is of the same order when the influence of other factors has been discounted in the latter case. Furthermore, overseas-qualified GPs have to make more job applications, even though they tend to have higher qualifications than British-qualified GPs.

GPs who came to the UK in early years, particularly up to 1959, tend to have found their present job more easily than those who came in more recent years. However, this finding is much less firmly established than the parallel one for hospital doctors because the number of GPs who came to the UK recently is rather small, and those who came up to 1959 (who definitely made fewer applications than the rest) are also an ethnically distinct group, containing a large number of doctors from continental Europe.

IX Findings from Informal Interviews at Hospitals

The detailed analysis of the survey findings which has been presented in the preceding chapters raised certain questions without answering them. For example, the survey shows that overseas-qualified doctors are much less likely than the British-qualified to be employed in teaching districts, but it does not show exactly why this is so. Again, it is clear from the survey that while a majority of overseas-qualified doctors progress at broadly the same rate as British doctors, some have severe difficulties and progress much more slowly, but it is not clear what are the basic reasons for the relative success of the one group as against the serious difficulties of the other; a difference in command of English does not seem to be the whole explanation. Answers to questions such as these cannot be given wholly within the rigorous but limited perspective of the survey findings.

We have tended to discuss these findings in the context of a simplified and schematic view of how things are done (for example, how medical staff are recruited or how doctors look for jobs) and of how people think (for example, about cultural differences and discrimination). The findings from our informal investigations within hospitals provide a more finely drawn context within which some of the survey findings can be better understood; they also help to answer some of the questions raised but not answered by the survey.

These informal investigations were carried out at two teaching hospitals (one in London and one outside London), three general hospitals (one in the Midlands and two in the North of England), two psychiatric hospitals (one in London and one in the Midlands), one geriatric hospital in London, and one psychiatric and geriatric hospital in the North of England. These 'hospitals' were sometimes in fact groups of hospitals whose administration was closely linked, and sometimes units within a larger group. At each one, informal interviews were carried out with British and overseas-qualified doctors at different levels, and where appropriate within different specialties. Where possible, administrative staff were also interviewed. Our conclusions are based on a total of about 100 interviews.

Unlike the survey, these informal investigations were not based on a sample (either of doctors or of hospitals) which is known to be representative. The only constraints applied when selecting hospitals were that each of a number of types of hospitals, and each of a number of regions, should be covered. The selection of doctors to be interviewed within hospitals was subject to many pressures which could lead to biasses. For example, among British consultants, those who were friendly to overseas doctors, or those who were hostile, might be especially likely to volunteer to be interviewed. In any case, the numbers are too small for the sample to be representative in the statistical sense. It is not appropriate, therefore, to treat the findings as a statistical source, but rather to use them as a source of insights which stand to be confirmed by more general facts or arguments, or by information from elsewhere — for example, from our own survey. We have presented the findings from these informal interviews in two parts. The first part deals with selection and training procedures and experiences and the second with the attitudes of overseas-qualified doctors and of British-qualified consultants and doctors.

PART 1   SELECTION AND TRAINING OF HOSPITAL DOCTORS

Recruitment, selection and job search
Most of the difficulties of overseas-qualified doctors lie in finding an appropriate sequence of junior hospital jobs and thereby gaining access to the training and experience for which they came to the UK. These are difficulties which they share to some extent with British-qualified doctors and which spring, to a large extent, from the general properties of the British system for the employment and training of junior hospital doctors. It is, therefore, important to consider this wider context.

In the British system, postgraduate medical training is conceived of as learning on the job and from informal contact with accomplished doctors, with a few elements of more formal instruction added from time to time. This kind of system is not universal; in fact, the approach in other countries such as USA and Canada could be caricatured as formal instruction with a few added elements of practical experience. The British system of learning on the job may well be the best one, but it is bound to lead to a tension between training and service objectives. At a local level, and in the short term, the objectives of training junior doctors well and providing a good service to patients may not coincide. Training objectives can be given greater priority to the extent that hospitals plan within a longer time scale, and to the extent that the activities of individual hospitals are linked to one another and to a planning system at regional and national levels. Although considerable progress has been made in this direction, there are still many hospitals where the immediate demands of the work to be done prevail over the training needs of junior doctors, and where these doctors consequently learn relatively little.

What is important for the present discussion, however, is not the training value of a particular job, but the way in which a junior doctor's total training programme is put together from a succession of jobs. Hospital doctors remain junior for at least seven years. During this time they need to gain experience of a number of different types of medicine. In most cases, these different kinds of experience will not all be available within the same hospital, although this will depend to some extent on the specialty and, of course, on the hospital. Thus, junior doctors will generally have to move about from one hospital to another, and certainly from one job to another, in order to obtain appropriate training and experience.

The current British system expects the junior doctor for the most part to put together his own training programme. In recent years, however, there has been an increase in the number of rotating posts at senior house officer and registrar level, and there is a set of training programmes for senior registrars (known as Higher Professional Training) which covers the final two to four years of a junior doctor's training.

A second important feature of the present system is the spheres of influence of teaching hospitals, partly formalised, partly informally understood, which help them to ensure a suitable succession of training posts for their own graduates. A third, and more subtle, factor is the placing of junior doctors in posts through the influence and connections of their consultants or other senior doctors with whom they have come in contact.

These factors tend to promote continuity of training and a suitable succession of jobs for those junior doctors who have got onto the bus at the first stop, while they tend to limit the opportunities for those who try to get on later. The three factors all represent limitations on the degree of open competition for junior hospital posts. In the case of the rotating posts, the different jobs that make up the rotation cease to be separately available and are allocated instead to those who have got past the first entry point. As to the spheres of influence of teaching hospitals and the 'placing' of junior doctors in posts through informal contacts, these have the effect of limiting open competition for jobs that are apparently available on the open market. They can, at the same time, be seen as semi-formal or informal systems for providing some continuity of training in a suitable succession of jobs for certain doctors, especially graduates of British medical schools. Whatever the advantages of such informal systems, they are bound to lead to inequities when there is a large influx of doctors from overseas.

Rotating posts

Perhaps the most important method currently used of providing both continuity and variety of training is through the creation of rotating posts by groups of hospitals acting jointly. This system is particularly well-developed for senior registrars, but there are also substantial numbers of rotating posts at registrar and senior house officer level. The Midland Area Training Scheme for senior registrars in anaesthesia can be cited as an example. The following is an extract from the official booklet describing the scheme.

'The Midland Area Training Scheme is a scheme aimed at providing a totally integrated training programme for senior registrars. The scheme includes all senior registrars within the Birmingham Region and those working in the United Birmingham Hospitals . . . . Rotation through the various hospitals is based primarily on trainees' needs, and there is free interchange between the United Birmingham Regional Hospital Board, because all appointments are joint appointments. In addition, the senior registrars receive an honorary appointment of a clinical tutorship to the University Department. After a period of time at the initial hospital to which the senior registrar is first appointed, recommendations are made that any individual trainee should rotate to another hospital in the Region (rotation is normally at the end of one year, and thereafter on an annual basis), if that particular hospital could satisfy the individual's training deficiencies . . . . It is anticipated that within three years of joining the Midland Area Training Scheme, a senior registrar would be ready to take up a consultant post.'

Schemes of this kind apply to one part only of a junior doctor's training; for senior registrars, they are universal, but at lower levels they are patchy. This creates a class distinction between the (desirable) rotating posts and the non-rotating ones (which are less desirable). In the informal investigations we found that some overseas doctors thought it was difficult or impossible for them to be accepted for rotating posts. For example, an Indian doctor interviewed at a teaching hospital outside London where he was registrar in neurosurgery (not on rotation) said that it was 'difficult — absolutely impossible — for an Asian doctor to get into a rotating job . . . . In this town there are no coloured chaps in rotating jobs'. This was certainly an exaggeration, but unfortunately we do not have evidence from the survey about the penetration of overseas doctors into rotating posts. We know that more than one-quarter of senior registrars are overseas-qualified, and all senior registrar posts are rotating and form part of a training system. How far overseas doctors succeed in getting into rotating posts at senior house officer and registrar level we do not know.

The spheres of influence of teaching hospitals

At the London teaching hospital where we carried out interviews, a carefully formalised system had been devised for placing graduates from the medical school in pre-registration house officer posts in the teaching hospital itself, in one of the other hospitals in the same Health District, or in one of the large number of hospitals in the region with which the teaching hospital had a 'special relationship'. The system takes into account how well the student passed out in his year and his preferences as between the house officer posts available.

The teaching hospital continues to look after its own graduates after their pre-registration year, principally by offering them jobs in the hospital itself or elsewhere in the district, but also by helping them into suitable jobs elsewhere. At senior house officer (SHO), registrar and senior registrar levels, jobs are advertised in the British Medical Journal (BMJ) although they are also posted on the appointments notice board in the hospital grounds. On the whole, SHO posts are filled by St. Jude's[1] graduates, but not invariably. For SHO casualty jobs the majority of candidates have usually just become registered, and about half usually are from overseas, especially from India and Pakistan. Those shortlisted would normally be from St. Jude's or other London teaching hospitals, unless an overseas candidate 'had something special about him'. According to an Indian consultant in this hospital:

> 'In this specialty when jobs are advertised at SHO and registrar level, for every home graduate there are four or five overseas applicants, mainly from the Indian sub-continent. The bulk are not shortlisted. It is not prejudice against them, it is because they are not known. I have difficulty explaining to Indian doctors that it is very much an old boys' network in an institution like ours. Your own graduates do and should get priority. Then there is the next category for shortlisting: someone rings up from another London teaching hospital and says one of the candidates is a nice chap. The third category is the friends of those who have been at St. Jude's. They increasingly write in to say in six months or a year they will be finishing their existing post and will there be any vacancies; when the time comes, as they are vouched for by St. Jude's or ex-St. Jude's doctors, they will probably be shortlisted.'

The implication is clearly that a graduate of St. Jude's can normally expect to be offered a succession of junior posts within his own teaching hospital, or at similar hospitals where his consultant's recommendation will be needed. In fact, an anaesthetics consultant at St. Jude's pointed out that four recently vacant senior house officer posts had been filled by four St. Jude's graduates after seven St. Jude's graduates had been shortlisted. This particular consultant had himself left his own teaching hospital before moving up to senior house officer and had, as a result, experienced considerable difficulty in finding a suitable job at this level.

At the teaching hospital which we investigated outside London, the tendency to fill posts with the hospital's own graduates seemed much less strong. Some informants denied that there was any such tendency, while

---

1 Fictitious names for hospitals and individuals are used throughout this chapter.

others thought that there was, but that it only operated at the margin.

The importance of these spheres of influence cannot be accurately assessed without carrying out special surveys of the staff of key teaching hospitals and associated hospitals to find out what proportion of the medical staff at different levels is made up by graduates of a given teaching hospital, and how far these hospitals do try to ensure that their graduates obtain a suitable succession of training jobs. Where they cannot offer a suitable job within the teaching hospital itself, or within another teaching hospital with which they have links, they probably try to fix up a job elsewhere.

This was certainly the opinion of a British consultant in general medicine whom we interviewed at a general hospital in the Midlands. When he was asked 'Why do overseas doctors generally find it hard to get a post in general medicine?' he replied 'One reason is that individual consultants often have links with a teaching hospital, and they get staff from their contacts with them'. An Indian consultant in psychiatry at another hospital said that 'at SHO level very few jobs in good hospitals are available to foreign doctors because such hospitals have arrangements to take the output of particular medical schools'. We have already pointed out that informal 'systems' of this kind have positive benefits: they help to ensure an orderly succession of training jobs for graduates of British medical schools (even if they help to preserve any 'pecking order' that may exist between these schools). However, when large numbers of overseas-qualified doctors are mixed into a system of this kind, inequities must immediately ensue. The 'system' acts to protect the training prospects of British graduates (who have patrons within it) but does not especially protect graduates from other countries (who have no patrons in this country).

Informal networks

The degree of formality involved in recruiting and appointing hospital doctors varies according to the seniority of the post. In the case of consultants, there is always a large appointment committee containing representatives of various different interests, and the whole procedure is highly formalised. This applies less to the more junior appointments. The following is a consultant's account of arrangements for appointing anaesthetists at a general hospital in the Midlands.

> 'When we advertise an SHO post we rarely see a white applicant, with the exception of Australians. We typically get ten applicants, but most of these will have applied for several or many other jobs at the same time. We normally invite four of these to an interview and two turn up. In the case of SHOs, I do the appointments myself with no committee and without consulting anyone else. In the case of registrars, there is an appointments committee at area level. It includes, for example, a lay member of the AHA, an administrator

from the AHA and the relevant consultant from the hospital. The consultant does the shortlist while the committee does the interviewing and makes the final appointment. The senior registrars are appointed in Birmingham by a regional committee (of the Midlands Area Training Scheme). I sit on the committee, and members state which candidates should be shortlisted.'

Here we have three kinds of procedure, neatly graded in terms of formality, from appointment by an individual consultant, through shortlisting by the consultant with appointment by a hospital committee, to shortlisting and appointment by a regional committee. There seem to be considerable local variations in the procedures followed, at any rate for senior house officer and registrar posts, but the pattern of increasing formality for the more senior posts seems to be common. A single consultant often has a large influence, or exclusive control, in the appointment of senior house officers, and to a lesser extent, registrars. We can quote as another example a psychiatric and geriatric hospital in the North of England.

'SHO jobs are advertised in the BMJ (or in the internal hospital bulletin) about four months before the post is expected to become vacant. When applications are received, the files go to the consultant with the most seniority in the specialty . . . This consultant alone has the job of seeing all the applications, and deciding who is to be shortlisted . . . . . The interview panel is made up of the consultant concerned and one of the hospital administrators. The procedure for registrars is much the same as for SHOs. There used to be a lay member of the authority on the selection panel but it proved too difficult to arrange convenient dates, so this has been dropped.'

From the fact that arrangements are often fairly informal and that a single consultant often has a very large say in certain appointments we might expect that the system is not completely open and that a doctor known to the consultant would often be placed in a junior post. From the career histories of doctors whom we informally interviewed it is clear that they did in fact often find their junior posts through personal contacts or recommendations. For example, one St. Jude's graduate whom we spoke to was allocated a house officer job not at St. Jude's but at one of the hospitals with which St. Jude's has a special relationship. At this hospital was a consultant physician who also worked at a third hospital nearby. The young doctor next got a house officer physician job at the third hospital. 'I made the arrangement myself through the consultant who worked in both hospitals, so although they did advertise the job, it was a formality'. Overseas-qualified doctors may also be able to make use of these informal networks, as can be seen from the early history of this senior registrar in anaesthetics at St. Jude's:

'I began my internship in Bombay but came to England in 1969 to join my husband and other members of my family. My husband was

157

a registrar in obstetrics and gynaecology at a hospital in Newtown and he arranged for me to start there. My first job was as a house officer in surgery for nine months, then I was an SHO in obstetrics and gynaecology for six months. The consultant anaesthetist suggested that I might like to try that specialty. I became an SHO in anaesthetics, and found I liked it very much, so I have stayed in the field. After eighteen months I became a registrar. All the house officer and senior house officer posts were offered to me, and not advertised; the registrar post was advertised, but I had been assured that I would get it.'

It is quite clear from this kind of history that once established in a hospital, a doctor who is liked and respected will tend to be offered a succession of jobs there (even though the hospital may go through the formality of advertising the posts). Of course, not all doctors will be fortunate enough to find themselves in hospitals in which they can gain the whole range of experience which they require.

An Australian senior registrar in rheumatology at St. Jude's provides another example of 'placing':

'I applied for the St. Jude's senior registrar post, advertised in the BMJ, while I was still at home, on the recommendation of another Melbourne registrar who had been at St. Jude's two years previously. It was arranged informally before I came — I doubt if I would have come otherwise. My boss met at a conference the man who was the existing holder of the post, and they fixed it up between them.'

This is how a registrar in the same department got his present job:

'I was lucky enough to come directly to the St. Jude's job. Some nine months before I was due to come to England, the head of the St. Jude's unit passed through New Zealand and said they might well have a job for me when I arrived.'

An Asian consultant geriatrician, describing an earlier part of his career, said 'My boss fixed me up at Birmingham as senior registrar in a rotating post'. We visited a large psychiatric hospital in London where training opportunities were generally good because most posts were rotating, the two other legs of the rotation being a teaching hospital and a district general hospital. Here, two of the doctors that we spoke to had found their posts (desirable ones within the field of psychiatry) by informal means.

'I took TRAB and in November 1976 did a clinical attachment at Pathways (a London teaching hospital). I had been assigned to a hospital in Oxford through DHSS, but I wrote to a few London hospitals and was offered the attachment at Pathways. In January 1977 I joined the rotating scheme as an SHO, becoming a registrar after three months.'

'When I came to England I first of all took courses at St. John's while preparing myself for TRAB, which I failed the first time but passed in July 1977. Then I worked with Professor Jones at Pathways for two months, on a voluntary basis as "honorary clinical assistant". After that, Professor Jones wrote to the GMC[2] and said that a clinical attachment wasn't necessary. I joined the rotation scheme in November 1977.'

Each of these doctors initially got into Pathways Hospital, a London teaching hospital, without having an appointment of the usual type. The first doctor bypassed the system for the allocation of clinical attachments, the second somehow became known to a professor who allowed the young doctor to work with him for a short time without pay. In both cases, the young doctors, having made themselves known within the teaching hospital, were offered rotating posts in psychiatry without having to apply for them formally.

A final example of the workings of informal networks is provided by the anaesthetics department of a general hospital in the Midlands already referred to. Here the head of the department had sole responsibility for appointments at SHO level. He tended to use this power to help young doctors whom he knew, or in whom he had confidence for some reason. For example, the wife of one of the registrars in anaesthetics had been helped: 'My wife is also working at this hospital. She spoke to Dr. Fogarty who offered a job here; at least, the job was advertised, and there were four candidates, but actually she was offered the job from the beginning.'

Another registrar in the same department explained how she had found her present job as follows: 'When I knew that my husband was coming to this area I went to see Dr. Fogarty to see if there were any jobs available, and he said he would give me a job when one became available. Within six weeks Dr. Fogarty did offer me a job.'

The same two doctors also used informal networks at earlier stages of their careers:

'I did my clinical attachment in Shrewsbury, and then six months in casualty in the same hospital, because I could not get an anaesthetics job at the time. But this job in casualty was good experience, and I enjoyed it. Then I did get an anaesthetics job in the same hospital, and I stayed in it for a year. While I was doing the casualty job I did not make applications for anaesthetics jobs elsewhere, but instead waited until a suitable job became available at the same hospital.'

'On coming to Britain I had a clinical attachment at Selly Oak. After that I became SHO at Southmead (a large general hospital in the Midlands). I found this job through Dr. Prince, who was my consul-

---

2 This seems to be a mistake, as the GMC would not be the appropriate body.

tant on the clinical attachment. What happened was that the SHO at Southmead went to Selly Oak as a registrar, while I went to fill the SHO post at Southmead, so they did a swap.'

From the way in which doctors talk about finding jobs, which is illustrated by these examples, it is clear that informal networks are an important factor. The examples also show that overseas doctors do benefit from these networks. Generally speaking, however, doctors who have trained in the UK will tend to have a better repertoire of networks on which to rely when they are looking for a job, so that the use of these networks will tend to work to the advantage of the British-qualified.

It may also be that overseas doctors, or some of them, tend to go about looking for a job in a more formal way than British doctors, and do not make so much use of informal networks that might be available to them, because they do not fully understand 'how these things are done' in the UK. For example, it may be quite usual for a British doctor to approach a consultant to ask if any opportunities are available in his department, or to ring up the consultant before applying for a post that is advertised to find out more about it and make himself known, or to cast around for connections or acquaintances who are ready to contact the consultant to 'put in a good word'. Overseas doctors may be unable to use this kind of technique, or may use it inappropriately, or may think of it as unacceptable canvassing. This is one of the universal disadvantages of the newcomer.

Criteria of selection
When filling junior posts, we have seen that consultants quite often appoint doctors who are known to them through informal networks. This is a reliable method of minimising risk. However, formal methods are also regularly used for junior appointments, and where they are, it becomes necessary to assess the relative merits of competing candidates according to some set of explicit or implicit criteria. This is easier where the post is more senior than where it is more junior, because applicants for more senior posts have done more on the basis of which they can be assessed. In the case of applicants for a registrar or senior registrar post, for example, a number of criteria can be applied on the basis of the written applications, at the shortlisting stage. Relevant factors would be the examination record, length of experience in particular specialties and subspecialties, the amount of experience, if any, in teaching hospitals or other well-regarded hospitals, and the time taken to reach the present point in the career structure. Subsequently, the choice among those shortlisted may be made on the basis of rather more subjective criteria, such as the quality of written references, the responses to informal telephone enquiries to the applicants' present consultants, and the impression created at interview.

In the case of applicants for more junior posts there is much less to go on. The MB or equivalent is a pass or fail examination, although special distinctions, prizes and so on are awarded, and graded results may be available internally within the teaching hospital. A doctor applying for a hospital job one or two years after passing the MB cannot be expected to have taken any postgraduate examination or to have done anything else to distinguish himself particularly (in medicine). The selection from among the shortlisted candidates is likely to be much influenced by references and personal recommendations, and by the impression created at the interview.

In the case of junior posts, therefore, because criteria of selection are hard to come by, the particular medical school attended is bound to be given some weight. It is in this light that most candidates tend to regard a preference for British-qualified at the expense of overseas-qualified doctors. Although few consultants have a detailed knowledge of the nature or standards of basic medical training in particular countries, still less at particular medical schools,[3] it is widely believed by British consultants that basic medical training at most medical schools in India, Pakistan and many Middle Eastern countries is inferior — probably markedly inferior — to that provided in the UK. This view may seem to be sanctioned by a system which denied full registration to doctors who qualified in these countries. Their qualifications were not 'recognised' for the purpose of full registration. Thus, a consultant who has a preference for British-qualified applicants for junior posts nearly always believes that this is justified by a difference in the value of the basic medical qualifications. This may or may not be a rationalisation of an ethnic or racial prejudice. In any case, it seems like a rational criterion, where good criteria are hard to find.

The basic training provided in white anglophone countries is generally thought to be superior to that provided in countries such as India and Pakistan; thus, ethnic and racial differences tend to coincide with alleged differences in the value of basic training. Country of qualification, therefore, is quite openly used as a criterion of selection.

Some finer distinctions between countries are sometimes made. There are some suggestions from our informal interviews that Egyptian basic training is considered by some to be better than that available in most other Arab countries, and also that Egyptians progress more quickly within the NHS than other Arabs. Unfortunately we cannot test this through the survey, since in the statistical treatment we have had to group all doctors from Arab countries together. Another example of an idea about a particular country came from a consultant geriatrician in London who strongly preferred Sri Lankan doctors to other Asians on the ground that the basic training in Sri Lanka was much better than in India. This consultant showed the courage of his convictions by filling his department with Sri Lankan doctors. Generally speaking, however,

---

3 Typically, consultants divide medical schools into very broad categories such as British, white Commonwealth, Indian sub-continent/Arab, and continental Europe.

preferences for doctors from particular countries are not usual, and knowledge of particular medical schools abroad is very rare.

Little weight is generally attached to experience gained in the country of origin, not necessarily because consultants doubt the value of such experience, but because they are not in a position to evaluate it. This goes a long way towards explaining why most migrant doctors start at senior house officer level in this country regardless of their previous experience in the country of origin. It also explains why overseas doctors have their greatest difficulties in finding the first job in the UK, and why the number of applications made tends to decrease for each successive job in this country.

The importance of command of English, as a criterion for deciding between overseas-qualified doctors, is hard to assess. At the shortlisting stage there is little reliable information about the applicant's English, although letters of application may vary to some extent in literacy, or more plausibly in the command that they show of slight socio-literary nuances. For example, doctors may respond unfavourably to a letter which ends 'Thanking you', as letters of application from Indians often do. However, examination of actual written applications suggests that they do not form a basis for rationally assessing the applicants' command of English. At a personal interview, command of English can, of course, be assessed, although consultants do not represent it as the most important criterion. On the other hand, when they make judgements of the applicants' other qualities, such as their medical skill or general intelligence, they may be mainly responding to how well they can talk about medicine and other subjects, or in other words to the standard of their spoken English.

The criteria of selection applied after personal interviews are, of course, very hard to define. One of our informants, a consultant, said that applicants would be judged at interview on 'manner, comportment, speech and accent'. On this view of the matter, the interview is a test of certain specific social skills and habits; these skills and habits are, of course, ones which a British doctor has had more opportunity to acquire than an overseas doctor. But these interviews may also have something in common with viva voce medical examinations: that is, the ability to talk around a medical problem may be tested. On this score, it was emphasised to us time and time again, British doctors have an enormous advantage, because they have practised a certain analytical approach to problems that is expected, whereas doctors who trained elsewhere are more likely to recapitulate textbook knowledge that is not strictly relevant.

Another criterion applied at interviews, which is related to the others, is compatability: Is this someone with whom I can work? The importance of this factor was nicely summarised by an informant who was talking about the appointment of one of his consultant colleagues.

'I don't feel that race is an important factor at all in medicine — it never has been. However, there are a lot of intangibles in appointing a consultant, and one has to consider that the person you appoint will be someone you will be working with very closely day after day. The decision is taken on the basis of credentials, and what one thinks of the applicant when one meets him, and how he "presents" at the actual interview: references are only taken up just before the interview or even after it and are of minor importance compared with these other things. In the case of the appointment of my colleague, Dr. Gupta, there were four people shortlisted, all Asians. . . . During the period before the interviews, three Manchester consultants phoned me up and said in one way or another that Dr. Gupta was "a very good colleague".'

'A very good colleague' seems to be the critical phrase and feeling.

The explanation of exceptional difficulties

At the beginning of this chapter we pointed out two questions which were raised but not answered by the survey findings. The first was why a comparatively small proportion of overseas-qualified doctors have found jobs in teaching hospitals. From the findings of the informal interviews it has already become plain that this is probably largely because the teaching hospitals have well-developed methods of looking after their own graduates which must work to the disadvantage of graduates from elsewhere. The second question raised was why some overseas doctors have exceptional difficulties, and in particular make very large numbers of applications before finding a job, while the majority progress at much the same rate as British doctors, and find jobs fairly easily. The answer to this second question is less straightforward.

It is best to focus attention on selection for the first or second job in the UK. In theory, it might be suggested that the sharp differences between the fortunes of different overseas doctors at this stage correspond to equally sharp differences in their medical or linguistic competence. On reflection, however, this seems most unlikely. As regards linguistic competence, among those doctors who have had extreme difficulties are some whose English is (now) good. In any case, the evidence suggests that overseas doctors have a rather uniformly mediocre standard of English on arrival (but that command of English tends to improve very markedly with every year that a doctor stays in this country). Thus, differences in command of English are unlikely to explain differences in the level of initial difficulties. As regards medical competence, there may indeed be sharp differences between different overseas doctors, but it is hard to see how selection committees can tell from the written applications of newly arrived doctors which are above and which below average. Yet the doctors who make large numbers of applications before finding a job are rarely offered an interview. Large numbers of consultants and selection committees concur in deciding not to shortlist them. At first sight they appear to be applying a common set of criteria, on the basis of the written applications alone, which relate to the doctors' competence; but it is hard to see what criteria would produce such a consistent result.

In fact, there are few criteria of any kind, whether or not relating to doctors' actual competence, which would lead to the continual rejection of a particular group, and which selection committees would be likely to apply. We have seen that consultants and selection committees have little detailed knowledge of particular medical schools in India, Pakistan or Middle Eastern countries and would therefore be most unlikely to prefer doctors from particular schools. We have also seen that they rarely favour doctors from particular countries within the Asian/Arab group. We have further seen that little if any weight is attached to experience gained in the country of origin. Even if large variations in language competence were important in this context (we have argued earlier that they are not) they would not generally be visible from the written applications. This leaves very little by which consultants are able to distinguish between newly arrived overseas doctors in any way at all.

Because there are few criteria that could be applied so as to lead to the consistent rejection of certain applicants when looking for their early jobs in the UK, we are thrown back on the suggestion that the important factor is strategies of job search rather than criteria of selection. There are also positive reasons for thinking that this is so. From the informal interviews, we found that the doctors who made very large numbers of applications were generally determined to find a job in general medicine or general surgery, or occasionally in some other popular specialty. They did not find a job by informal methods, for example, through the recommendation of the consultant with whom they did their clinical attachment. (This could be through ignorance of 'how these things are done' or because their first consultant formed a low opinion of them.) These doctors tended to persist with the strategy of trying to find a job in a popular specialty as a first step, even though they were rejected a very large number of times. They tended to make applications indiscriminately for jobs which they knew nothing about, in hospitals that they had never heard of, and they did not try to make themselves known beforehand at the hospitals to which they were applying. When they reluctantly decided to look for a job in a less popular specialty (such as geriatrics or psychiatry) they were usually offered one very quickly.

The overseas doctors who have not had serious difficulties tend either to have chosen a less popular specialty at the outset, or to have adopted more flexible strategies for finding a suitable job in a popular specialty. Those who initially decided to go, for example, into geriatrics, psychiatry or anaesthetics, have not generally experienced difficulties. Among those who have gone into general medicine or general surgery, some found their first job through the recommendation of the consultant with whom they did their clinical attachment, or more indirectly by using his contacts. Others decided to take a job in a good hospital although it was not what they wanted, but then looked out for suitable opportunities in that hospital, where they were known. Others somehow made personal contacts with a few consultants who might have suitable jobs to offer.

To some extent, the difference in the fortunes of these two groups may be related to a difference in ability or accomplishment based on the judgement of the consultants with whom they come into contact. Those who seem more accomplished will, for example, be more likely to be placed in a job by the consultant with whom they do their clinical attachment. To a greater extent the different fortunes are probably a consequence of the different strategies adopted by the two groups of doctors. This is not to imply that the more flexible type of strategy is necessarily the 'correct' one. A doctor who has come to the UK to become a plastic surgeon may be right, up to a point, to persist for a long time before accepting a post outside surgery, since he might find it difficult to get back into surgery later. However, strategies inflexibly adopted may have been unrealistic from the outset. Only 28 per cent of adult migrants in the survey had information from an authoritative British body about training and working opportunities before they came to this country. It would not be surprising if among the remaining 72 per cent there were some who failed to adjust their plans to reality.

It seems likely that newly arrived doctors from the Indian subcontinent or Middle Eastern countries will nearly always be rejected when formally applying for good training posts in general medicine or general surgery. The doctors who have got into extreme difficulties may be the ones who did not realize that this is so, and who were not lucky or outstanding enough to be offered a job through some informal network. This suggests that there is a need for a more structured training programme, or at the least, for more guidance, a theme which will be expanded in the final chapter.

The special case of geriatrics
We have seen from the survey that a relatively high proportion of overseas-qualified doctors are in geriatrics and that this is seldom from choice. The informal investigations confirm that it is rare for any doctor, whether British or overseas-qualified, to choose geriatrics freely at an early stage, and that most geriatricians originally intended to be general physicians.

The underlying reason for this is that geriatrics is not a specialty or sub-specialty in the usual sense. Ordinarily when doctors are said to specialise, this means that they acquire a specific body of knowledge and specific skills that are required for particular kinds of medical activity (such as surgery, laboratory work or radiodiagnosis) or for the treatment of a particular class of disorders (such as heart disease or mental illness). Geriatricians, by contrast are restricted to patients within a particular age group, who may have any disorder, requiring treatment from any of the specialties. A few disorders are characteristic of old people, but most

165

of the disorders of old people are ones from which younger people also suffer. The geriatrician is therefore a physician with a restricted clientele, rather than a specialist as such. The disadvantage of this position is that the more interesting and challenging cases may tend to be dealt with by specialists who have a more definite claim on them, so that the geriatrician is left with the chronic cases.

There is much discussion in the medical profession about the best way of organising the treatment of old people, and the systems of organisation which are currently most widespread are commonly thought to be unsatisfactory. We do not wish to add to this discussion, but merely to show that the brunt of any inadequacies falls on overseas-qualified doctors who have failed to achieve their objectives and find themselves in geriatrics by default. The career history of Dr Mujib illustrates this point.

Dr. Mujib, who comes from Bangladesh, qualified there in 1961, and worked as a hospital doctor there for twelve years, first in general medicine and then in chest medicine, reaching the grade of resident physician in 1973. At this stage, he got a scholarship from the World Health Organisation to spend four months of full time study in Czechoslovakia leading to a diploma in chest medicine. He then came to the UK, in June 1973, with the objective of becoming a member of the Royal College of Physicians (MRCP). After his clinical attachment, he applied for at least 100 jobs in general medicine, but did not succeed in getting one. Eventually he took a job in chest medicine (in which he had special experience and qualifications) as senior house officer. He stayed in this job for three years, and during this time he tried and failed to pass Part 1 of the MRCP several times. He then tried again to find a job (still as senior house officer) in general medicine, but again failed after making about 100 applications and only once being offered an interview. He therefore decided to get a job in geriatrics, and found a senior house officer post at his present hospital after making only two or three applications; after three months he moved up to registrar grade. At the time when we spoke to him he was waiting for the result of his fourth attempt at Part 1 of the MRCP. He said he was feeling very depressed.

'I never wanted to be a geriatrician, and I still don't want to be. It is just that I can't get a job in general medicine, and geriatrics provides some of the relevant experience for the MRCP, although it's second best . . . . I want to go back, but there are so many uncertainties. It depends on many factors. I never expected to stay as long as five years, but I have done so. If I don't get the MRCP I won't get a job here, I don't know what I will do. In order to get Part 2, I need to get experience of medicine in this country, I need to see patients, to see the diseases here, in this land, because Part 2 is practical bread-and-butter medicine of England, and not that of other countries in the world. One must have some fundamental training in this country. I respect the system here. It is a good system. But I have been unable to get the training that I need.'

Access to training

The junior doctor's access to training depends on whether or not he is able to put together a good training programme, consisting of an appropriate succession of jobs stretching over a five to seven-year period, and on the nature and amount of training available within each particular job in the sequence. We have already discussed why it is more difficult for overseas than for British-qualified doctors to build up an appropriate sequence of jobs. The nature and amount of training available within particular jobs deserves further discussion.

An attempt was made in the survey to assess junior doctors' access to specific training and training facilities in their present jobs through a series of factual and attitudinal questions. Generally, these questions showed little difference between British and overseas-qualified junior doctors, but this could be because they did not distinguish finely enough between different factors, and in particular, between different kinds of specific training activity. At least eight relevant kinds of activity can be distinguished.

(a) Formal courses outside the hospital, for example at universities or teaching hospitals. Some courses are full time over a short period, others on one morning, afternoon or evening per week over a longer period.

(b) Formal lectures within the hospital, given by a visiting speaker or by one of the consultants.

(c) Case conferences, in which a consultant or senior registrar presents a case which is then discussed by those present.

(d) Case conferences in which junior doctors as well as seniors may present a case for discussion.

(e) Journal clubs, at which a senior or junior doctor gives an account of an important journal article, which is then generally discussed by those present.

(f) Tuition given by consultants to junior doctors either individually or in small groups.

(g) Film shows organised by drug companies.

(h) Learning 'on the job'.

The first seven items on this list are forms of organised study (though item (g) is also a method of advertising) as opposed to learning 'on the job'. There may be important differences in the value of these various activities, and in their value to doctors with different backgrounds and at different stages of their careers. Doctors at prestigious institutions such as London teaching hospitals often consider that external courses are unnecessary for those whose basic medical education was a sound one. Overseas doctors tend to have much more faith in courses than the British-qualified, perhaps because they are aware of real gaps in their basic knowledge, perhaps because formal instruction is highly valued within the background from which they came.

Case conferences and journal clubs are generally thought to be more valuable than formal courses or lectures. They may be particularly valuable to Asian junior doctors where they give them an opportunity to present a case themselves and thus to develop a technique of presentation and analysis which is important in this country, for example, for viva voce examinations, but which they may not have practised at medical schools and hospitals in India and Pakistan.

We know from the survey that there is no difference between British and overseas-qualified doctors in the total amount of time spent in organised study of some kind, that is in any of the first seven kinds of activity listed. We do not know, however, which activities are of most value in any particular hospital or how far overseas doctors have access to, and make use of, those activities which could help them most.

Although doctors disagree about the value of different kinds of specific training activity, there is general agreement that the most important aspect of training is learning on the job. The opportunity for this kind of learning may vary widely from one job to another. What seems to be important is exactly how the consultant uses the available cases to teach the juniors (the use of the word 'teach' does not necessarily imply overt instruction or demonstration, but implies doing something that enables the juniors to learn). Because those involved tend to emphasise the elusive nature of this kind of learning, it is quite difficult to analyse what actually happens, and what doctors think ought to happen, but it is useful to set out some possibilities.

(i) The consultant performs a task while the juniors watch; the consultant makes appropriate comments and explanations, the juniors ask questions, are asked to tackle any problems that arise and put forward their own solutions.

(ii) The juniors help the consultant to perform the task, with comments, questions, explanations as before.

(iii) The juniors perform a task under the direct supervision of the consultant; that is, he watches, helps if the junior gets into difficulties, and engages in a dialogue as the work proceeds.

(iv) The consultant defines a task and tells the junior to perform it; the junior then performs the task without direct supervision, but may ask the consultant for help if he gets into difficulties.

(v) Cases are sorted into those to be dealt with by the consultant and those to be dealt with by the junior. The consultant is available to give advice or help to the junior, if required.

(vi) Cases are sorted (as in (v)) but the consultant is not usually available.

(vii) The junior deals with all cases, but may seek help or advice from the consultant.

(viii) The junior deals with all cases, and the consultant is not easily available to give help or advice. (This is not supposed to happen, but it may do in practice.)

A detailed study of medical training in hospitals would use some classification such as this one, and would seek to establish how many junior doctors receive how much 'training' of each type. This would be a substantial study in its own right, and we have not been able to carry it out, but certainly the indications from our informal investigations are that systems like (vi) (vii) or (viii) are fairly common; these are ways of working in which the junior doctors deal with all cases, or with some of them, normally without the help or advice of the consultant. Doctors tend to be more critical of past than of present jobs; they quite often describe past jobs in which they simply carried out (often routine) medical work without any kind of supervision or advice. According to a senior lecturer at St. Jude's: 'During the period before I came to St. Jude's I really had no teaching, no training, no guidance or advice at all . . . Once I had got to St. Jude's, I found that teaching was continuous— the consultants taught you as you saw cases instead of treating you as a dogsbody'. A more detailed account of a lack of supervision and advice was given by a woman doctor from Sri Lanka who first took a geriatric job in the UK after failing to find a job in general medicine. In this job:

'The training was really very good — the consultant was interested and concerned and spent considerable time teaching on ward rounds. In addition, there was an active postgraduate centre so I could keep up with general medicine to a certain extent. Then I was looking again for a general medicine job, and applied for 50-70 jobs. Finally I got an SHO post, but it was very unsatisfactory. It was a five-ward cottage hospital: two medical wards, two surgical, one paediatric. There were two part-time consultants who came in once a week each, but otherwise the other SHO and I were expected to run the hospital with no other medical help. I stayed in this post for one year. I trained myself. I was asked to stay on for another year but I wanted to get a registrar job. At an interview at another London hospital they said I was not qualified for a registrar post because I had been working so much on my own, but they agreed to try me as a locum registrar for three months; at the end of that period they would have to advertise the post but I would stand a good chance of getting it. Again, I was placed in a position of great activity and responsibility. There were far too many beds, four out-patient clinics, casualty duty every third day, and after a fortnight the consultant went off on leave for six weeks. As he didn't get on with his colleagues they wouldn't cover for him, so when I needed information I had to phone another hospital nearby.'[4]

---

4 The employing authority has a responsibility to ensure that there is always cover, but apparently did not do so in this case.

Some doctors think that it is only at teaching hospitals that good postgraduate training is available, but many others quote examples of good training at non-teaching hospitals.

'I can't speak highly enough of the training at St. Hilda's, which is small enough so that the consultants give personal attention, teaching and encouragement to the juniors. It is not that they don't have confidence in the juniors, but rather that they take their teaching role seriously. The whole schedule of the consultants is geared to a teaching relationship, not only on the ward rounds. For example, my consultant used to set aside an hour every Wednesday specifically to teach the junior doctors about such basic concepts as depression, anxiety, mood; and then during ward rounds on Thursdays he used to make a special point of discussing these in relation to individual patients.'

These examples show that there can be great variation between one hospital and another in the nature and degree of supervision and in the way in which work is organised. Of course, the experiences that doctors recounted to us were in the past, and systems may be improving considerably. At senior registrar level the training content of jobs is now effectively monitored. At more junior levels, efforts are being made to introduce a continuous monitoring of the training and supervision provided, with the sanction of withdrawing educational recognition from the post. We cannot say how effective these policies now are, because the information from our informal investigations relates to an earlier period. The impression created of that period is that what was meant by postgraduate teaching on the job and by the supervision of juniors was uncertain and open to widely different interpretations. Together with the inequality of resources between different areas and different specialties, this created the conditions in which there were bound to be sharp variations in the training value of different jobs. These sharp variations, combined with the absence of planned training programmes except at senior registrar level, are the conditions that ensure that among a disadvantaged group such as the overseas-qualified, there will be an important proportion who fail to obtain suitable training. Within the present system many doctors are trained very well indeed, because they do receive personal supervision from an experienced consultant while performing tasks, and engage in a continuous dialogue with the consultant about what they are doing; this must be an excellent way of learning. But it may also be easy for other doctors to receive no significant training at all.

PART 2   ATTITUDES OF INDIVIDUAL DOCTORS

In the course of the informal investigations we interviewed 43 Asian, Arab and African doctors. For these doctors — who are admittedly not necessarily representative of the wider population — we have a more sensitive and rounded description of attitudes than could emerge from the structured survey. This allows us to give a fuller account of overseas doctors' views of the difficulties they have encountered, and in particular, of their attitudes towards unequal treatment and discrimination.

In order to tackle the subject of unequal treatment in the survey, we had to devise a series of tightly worded questions which imposed on informants certain categories of thought.

The general drift of the findings from these questions was that most overseas doctors were convinced that they were not (as a group) treated equally when applying for hospital jobs; many thought this was the result of wrong judgements about the value of overseas qualifications and the competence of doctors from a different culture to practise in the UK. Comparatively few (18 per cent) thought that this kind of unequal treatment could be described as ethnic or racial discrimination, while about the same proportion thought they had themselves been victims of discrimination when applying for hospital jobs. When asked to say what made them think that unequal treatment occurred, nearly one-half of overseas doctors (44 per cent) gave answers which showed that they thought it was only to be expected (see Chapter VIII).

Attitudes of overseas doctors

In the informal interviews, informants were not necessarily asked specifically about unequal treatment or discrimination if these topics did not emerge naturally out of a discussion of their own careers and the position of overseas doctors in the UK. In practice, half of the overseas-qualified doctors interviewed (not including white anglophones) never mentioned anything that could be construed as unequal treatment or discrimination. For these doctors, the topic was not salient, although many of them would no doubt have said that unequal treatment occurred if they had been asked (as they would have been in the survey). They tended to be doctors with a relatively short experience in this country, or who had encountered few difficulties.

Whereas 44 per cent of overseas doctors in the survey seemed to think that unequal treatment was explicable, not many of those informally interviewed did so. This suggests that the survey informants who found unequal treatment understandable are mostly doctors for whom this issue is not of pressing importance, and who would not have mentioned it if (as in the informal interviews) they had not been specifically asked. Thus, it is probably more accurate to say that there is a large group of overseas doctors (approaching one-half) who are not strongly concerned about unequal treatment, than to say that these doctors draw attention to the rejection of their own group.

Whereas nearly half of overseas-qualified doctors in the survey thought that selection committees tend to reject overseas applicants because they wrongly put a lower value on their qualifications or because they wrongly considered they would be less competent to practise in the UK, a comparatively small proportion (18 per cent) agreed with the statement that 'they (the selection committees) discriminate on ethnic or racial grounds'. From the informal interviews, we can confirm that ethnic or racial discrimination is not a category of thought that overseas doctors commonly apply in this context; in fact, the term 'discrimination' was seldom, if ever, used in connection with unsuccessful job applications. However, this does not in the least imply that the unequal treatment is not condemned, or that it does not arouse feelings of bitter resentment on occasion. It is rather that the rejection of Asian (also Arab and African) doctors is not thought to spring exclusively or even primarily from racial or ethnic considerations, and the prejudices involved are thought to be specifically medical as well as connected with more general racial or ethnic stereotypes. The bias which nearly one-half of overseas doctors consider British consultants and selection committees to have is one which is articulated in terms of qualifications and competence rather than in terms of race and ethnic origin, hence the relatively small proportion of doctors who think that 'racial discrimination' occurs. Under the law, a systematic tendency to undervalue overseas qualifications or the competence of overseas doctors might well amount to racial or ethnic discrimination, but overseas doctors are not knowledgeable about the law, and this is not the category of thought which they spontaneously apply in this context. They may also hesitate to commit themselves (when talking to a white British interviewer) to a judgement which roundly condemns others and is humiliating to themselves.

We find from the informal interviews that where there is bitterness and resentment on the part of overseas doctors this is not focussed on complaints of unequal treatment of job applicants alone, but extends to other issues too, such as access to training and social relationships between white and coloured doctors. The doctors with the strongest feelings of this kind were Asians who had long experience of medical practice in the UK, and who had in some cases by now reached consultant status.

Specific examples

Dr. Bhaktia, who is now a consultant geriatrician, is an example. Dr. Bhaktia's attitude is shaped, to a large extent, by the great difficulties that he has faced in reaching his present position. In the nine years after his arrival in the UK he did nine different jobs in chest medicine and general medicine, none of which, he considers, offered him good training opportunities. Only at the end of this period did he pass Part 1 of the MRCP, after having made several previous attempts. He felt that he would not be able to pass Part 2 without having better clinical experience, and to this end he applied for a job as locum medical assistant in geriatrics in a teaching hospital. In 1967, he finally passed his Part 2 after doing this job for six months, and he believes that he managed to pass principally because he had finally gained access to suitable training (even though this was in geriatrics rather than general medicine). Dr.

Bhaktia feels very strongly that he did not gain access to the training for which he came to this country, and he believes that the doctors now coming are still not receiving adequate training in many cases.

Dr. Bhaktia's complaints about access to training are not based on any rigid or possibly unrealistic assumption that the standards of overseas doctors on arrival are generally the same as those of comparable British doctors. On the contrary, he concedes that the standards of overseas doctors may initially be lower in some ways, but argues from this that these doctors should be given full access to the best training so that they can improve. Thus, Dr. Bhaktia does not really blame consultants for preferring English graduates: 'their approach to patient care is better, more thoughtful and individual, less rigidly textbook in nature. But if overseas doctors are allowed into the country they should obtain the training which will help them develop this approach, and at present this is not done'.

A second reason for Dr. Bhaktia's bitterness is the difficulty that he encountered in gaining a consultant post after he had passed the MRCP. At this time, he had twelve interviews out of fifteen applications made, which he ascribes to the fact that his consultant was very well known and highly thought of. In eight out of the twelve cases when he was interviewed, no appointment was made, while in the other four cases a 'local candidate', that is, a British graduate, got the job. In four out of the eight cases where no appointment was made there was subsequent correspondence between his consultant and the selection committee. Two particular cases were mentioned in which the correspondence had been initiated by a member of the selection committee, in one case a senior physician, in the other an external assessor, and in both cases these committee members wrote to say that they objected to the failure to appoint Dr. Bhaktia, but had been unable to persuade their colleagues. Among the reasons given for not appointing him was that he had not held a senior registrar post in geriatrics, but he says that there were only three such posts in the country at the time. When he applied for his present consultant post, all eight candidates for two jointly advertised posts were overseas-qualified. One of the areas made no appointment, but 'one of those on the other panel was a British-qualified Indian woman, and she put her foot down and insisted on an appointment being made'. These experiences of being repeatedly rejected, as he sees it for no good reason, have made Dr. Bhaktia bitter. but it is still unclear whether he would accuse selection committees of 'ethnic or racial discrimination'. This is not the term that he uses, but he clearly considers that the repeated rejections were quite unjustified. He is also reacting to what he has heard about the experience of other people. For example, he claims that his wife, who is also Indian and a doctor, made 600 applications for jobs before obtaining a post in anaesthetics at a hospital where the consultant 'was known to prefer Indian ladies because they were more biddable'.

A third reason for Dr. Bhaktia's bitterness is that even though he has achieved consultant status he is still not accepted by English consultants at the hospital, who, he considers, are completely uninterested in any but the most superficial professional relationships with the overseas doctors.

There are considerable similarities in the experience and attitudes of Dr. Chahin, another Indian, who is a consultant paediatrician. Dr. Chahin came to the UK in 1955 and worked first for one year as a senior house officer in casualty and then for a second year at the same grade in surgery 'but with the promise of a medical job later' (which did not materialise). In these two jobs Dr. Chahin says there was no supervision, guidance or training of any kind, and no time off for reading; in the second job he was on call virtually without a break for three months continuously. Although he wanted a job in paediatrics, the best that he could get next was one in infectious diseases, which lasted for another year. However, in spite of these difficulties, Dr. Chahin passed the MRCP in 1958, only three years after coming to the UK. Because of his own early experience and what he has seen since, he is strongly critical of training provision for overseas doctors. He would favour a stiff selection at an initial entry point with a much more structured training programme thereafter.

> 'Of the Indian doctors in this country, about 50 per cent probably on arrival have potential to do well, given some encouragement. Some attempt should be made to make entrance more rigid, to weed out some of the other 50 per cent who have inadequate ability and education. Once the doctors are admitted, more emphasis should be placed on their training — it is useless to be in a peripheral hospital with such a work load that no progress can be made. Formal seminars and courses are not what is required at SHO level but rather more time and concern by the consultant in explaining and guiding.'

Dr. Chahin passed the MRCP relatively quickly and subsequently encountered fewer difficulties than Dr. Bhaktia in finding jobs. Nevertheless, he too had some difficulties in finding a consultant post, which brought home to him the importance of unequal treatment of overseas doctors. He had always planned to return to India, since he had not expected to be able to get a consultant post in the UK, but his own consultant insisted that he was 'consultant material', and this encouraged him to change his plans. He found his present job at the fifth attempt, but he had a number of discouraging experiences on the way. The most discouraging was a case where, he says, he had far better qualifications and experience than the other candidates; he learned 'on the grapevine' afterwards that his appointment had been supported by seven out of nine on the committee, but opposed by the other two, but that the seven supporters had not been prepared to 'make an issue of it'. The job was readvertised.

Dr. Chahin did not expect selection committees to be entirely without prejudice or bias. He thought that it was only natural that British-qualified doctors should receive preference even if they were slightly less able or well-qualified, but not if the gap was as wide as it had been on this occasion. Finding jobs up to registrar level was not difficult, he thought, but there was 'tremendous prejudice among English consultants' which made movement beyond that point difficult for overseas doctors.

Even after reaching consultant status, Dr. Chahin, like Dr. Bhaktia, certainly did not feel that he was accepted by the British consultants. He saw overseas doctors as being isolated within the hospital and left out either by accident or by design from the mainstream of hospital life. There was no place where consultants in different specialties could meet, and there was consequently a lack of contact, particularly at an informal level, between British and overseas-qualified doctors in the hospital. The overseas doctors felt rejected as a result. Dr. Chahin particularly mentioned that the merit awards[5] for consultants bred ill-feeling and resentment and that the various ethnic groups were not always properly represented on hospital committees.

The career of a third Indian consultant whom we interviewed, Dr. Vengat, might be regarded as wholly exceptional, in that he is now a consultant at a teaching hospital. Dr. Vengat first qualified as a doctor in India, but then came to Britain and immediately took the British MB examinations. He is, therefore, a British-qualified doctor who nevertheless had his basic training in India. Dr. Vengat speaks English perfectly, and as a young doctor was already well-qualified. As a junior doctor he had some difficulties, nevertheless, in getting suitable training jobs, although these difficulties were overcome, and he finally completed an impressive training programme. It was at this point, when he began to apply for consultant posts, that he encountered serious difficulties. He made 18 or 20 applications, and was shortlisted seven or eight times without success. He was beginning to become desperate and to apply for posts which his consultant thought were quite unsuitable. At this point, he was shortlisted for a consultant post by a selection committee which contained two doctors with whom he had previously worked — he had collaborated with one of them on a scientific paper. Through these contacts he found out how the committee had discussed his application. It emerged that the superintendent of the hospital flatly refused to appoint him, saying that the matron would not work with an Asian consultant. No appointment was made. Someone who heard about this case offered Dr. Vengat a locum job as consultant at his present hospital; he was later appointed a substantive consultant.

Dr. Vengat said that if he had had difficulties in finding a job as consultant in spite of the fact that 'my training had been first class, I had done all the very top jobs and had done research', then other overseas

---

5 There are four levels of merit award for consultants which are a supplement to the basic salary.

doctors with lesser qualifications and experience must have had still greater difficulties. Although the period of his greatest difficulties was ten years ago, he thinks that 'in some ways it is more difficult now'.

Dr. Vengat's case is particularly interesting because he was exceptionally well-qualified for a consultancy in a shortage specialty, because he is a person who appears to fit equally smoothly into British and Indian surroundings, and because he has always sought to join the British medical establishment rather than to fight it. He still had considerable difficulty in finding a consultant post. This leaves him with very ambivalent attitudes towards the medical establishment with which, in a sense, he identifies himself. On the one hand, he tends to defend the old boy network surrounding his own teaching hospital. On the other, he is very conscious of the difficulties of Indian and other overseas doctors less fortunate than himself, and he proposes various changes in the system to improve their training prospects. However, he advocates to them his own strategy of joining, or seeming to join, the system, rather than forming pressure groups which hope to change it from outside. By contrast, Dr. Bhaktia and Dr. Chahin, although consultants, still feel that they are outside in the cold, and do not believe that they will ever be accepted as members of the club.

The three Indian consultants whom we have quoted as examples vary widely from each other in the ease with which they have found jobs, passed examinations and progressed up the career ladder, in the degree to which they are assimilated to the English middle class and in the stance that they adopt as foreigners in the UK. Nevertheless, they have all encountered serious difficulties particularly in finding a consultant post and have come to the conclusion that the judgements of selection committees tend to be prejudiced against overseas doctors, although it is not at all clear that they think of this as a racial or even ethnic prejudice. All three consultants feel that there are serious inadequacies in the training available to many overseas doctors, and they are inclined to advocate rather general changes of policy to deal with this, such as the organisation of much more structured training programmes possibly combined with restriction of entry to doctors who pass a fairly rigorous selection procedure. Two of the three consultants feel that Indian doctors are essentially rejected and kept at a distance by the British medical profession, even when they become consultants; the third has successfully assimilated with the English middle class.

Doctors at the more junior level, who have spent a shorter period in the UK, are generally less likely to voice criticisms or to have feelings of bitterness and resentment, but where they do, they tend to make many of the same points. Dr. Ganesh, an Indian woman anaesthetist, has reached the grade of senior registrar after eight years in the UK without encountering enormous difficulties, and is now in a good rotating post. She recognised that she had few problems compared with many other overseas-qualified doctors, but mentioned that she had twice been rejected for jobs where she thought that the person chosen was not as good as she was (in both cases the successful applicant was British-qualified). She said: 'If I were to experience the same thing again I wouldn't be too upset: it's what I've come to expect.' Nevertheless, she feels that it is quite wrong that a British-qualified candidate should be preferred despite less good qualifications and experience, although 'everything is so subjective in an interview — it may be that personality comes into it.' Her own resentment at these two experiences of rejection she sees as a small indication of a more general feeling of frustration among Asian doctors at the difficulty of getting jobs even when they are apparently qualified for them. Apart from unequal treatment of Asian job applicants, she feels that there is a more general rejection of Asian doctors by the medical establishment, and a failure to move one inch to accommodate to them, even to the extent of learning to pronounce their names correctly, so that 'the rift becomes greater'. Like two of the Indian consultants whom we have quoted, Dr. Ganesh would like to see a stiff examination at the entry point for overseas doctors though she did not propose a structured training programme thereafter.

Training programmes and examination procedures

A Sri Lankan senior registrar in the same hospital put forward a different suggestion about the training programmes for overseas doctors. He felt that doctors who had come to the UK for training and who intended to return to the country of origin should be separated at the entry point from those who had come to make a permanent career in this country. Those who had come to the UK temporarily for training would be allocated to a series of 'attachments' rather than becoming part of the regular training hierarchy, while those who come to stay permanently should join the regular system. This suggestion is mentioned not because it is a practical one as it stands, but as a further illustration of the fact that many overseas (and British) doctors think that present arrangements for the training of overseas doctors are fundamentally unsound, and propose radical changes whose objective is to ensure that once allowed into the UK, doctors obtain the training for which they came.

The same doctor also illustrates a milder attitude towards unequal treatment. He has been looking for a consultant post for three or four years, but so far he has always been in competition with British-qualified applicants, one of whom has been appointed. He clearly feels that there is bias against overseas-qualified applicants for these posts, although he says that it is not specific discrimination against overseas doctors so much as the functioning of the old boy network. He is sure that 'a lot of pre-interview canvassing goes on' and that often it is probably quite clear who will get the post beforehand; British-qualified candidates are better able to use the relevant networks.

It has become generally known over the past few years, following the publication of statistics for a few specialties, that the pass rate of overseas-qualified entrants for membership and fellowship examinations is substantially lower than that of British-qualified entrants. This information is used by different doctors in different ways. One of the British consultants whom we interviewed argued from the examination results for his own specialty (which were privately rather than publicly available) that overseas-qualified doctors tended to be incompetent and slow to learn, and that it was therefore legitimate to exclude them from jobs and training, and to cultivate all British-qualified departments. The exactly opposite argument, of course, is that if pass rates are low among the overseas-qualified, then compensatory training programmes are required to bring them up to the required standard. We did not hear this argument being put up by overseas doctors, but we did encounter a third point of view : that it was bias in the examinations which was at least partly responsible for the low pass rates among the overseas-qualified.

Because parts of the fellowship and membership examinations are viva voce there is a real possibility of bias against candidates who manifestly belong to a different culture from the examiners. The issue is clouded by doubt as to what would, in any case, constitute a bias in these circumstances. It is important to realise (without cynicism) that no-one but the examiners can be sure what it is that they are trying to assess in oral examinations. A candidate might, for example, address himself to the clinical problems extremely well, but if he spoke with a thick accent the examiners might fail him on the ground that his patients would not be able to understand what he said. Whether or not this would be proper is unclear.

Two of our informants in particular were concerned about bias in the examinations. The first of these was Dr. Ganesh, the Indian woman anaesthetist whom we have already quoted. She said that there was a strong feeling among Asian doctors that there is deliberate discrimination in Part 2 of the membership and fellowship examinations. When she went for her Part 2 there were 80 candidates, of whom 20 passed, and 19 of these 20 were English (although Dr. Ganesh did not say so, in anaesthetics a high proportion of the candidates would have been overseas-qualified). This kind of ratio, said Dr. Ganesh, was what made people feel bitter, as well as the fact that people seemed to fail on a different part of the examination each time. She realized that this might be partly a matter of presentation techniques : she had consciously improved her own, which had probably helped her to pass Part 2. However, she did not think that presentation was the whole of the explanation.

The second doctor, who complained much more bitterly about examination bias, was also an anaesthetist. Dr. Patel concluded that there was a bias partly because of the discrepancy in pass rates (from unofficial rather than official statistics) and partly because of his own experience on a particular occasion. The essence of his view was that 'the local boys are tested on what they do know, whereas the overseas doctors are tested on what they don't know.' He claimed that a particularly high proportion of overseas doctors failed on the viva voce part of the examination, and that it was here that most of the bias occurred, although he thought that there was also bias in the marking of the essay part of the written examination.

Dr. Patel put the rather extreme view that examiners were actively hostile to overseas candidates and intentionally did not give them a chance to show what they knew. These very strong feelings could have been aroused by a serious misunderstanding that arose between himself and a group of examiners on one particular occasion because of a difference in expectations and unwritten understandings on the two sides; or, of course, it could have been true that these examiners were actively hostile to Dr. Patel. He generalised from this experience, saying that examiners pursued lines of questioning about trivial matters, particularly when the candidate became anxious and could not answer, and refused to switch to another topic where the candidate could not perform well on the one chosen.

The particular experience that Dr. Patel quoted was an interesting one. The examiners showed him a certain medical electronic gadget and asked 'What is in that box?' He could explain what the machine did, and what it was used for, but he could not say what was inside it, since it contained only electrical circuits, about which he did not know in detail. Although it was clear that he did not know how to tackle the question, the examiners persisted with it until Dr. Patel became thoroughly disconcerted and eventually failed. From this account it sounds as though Dr. Patel failed to recognise small socio-linguistic cues which would have told him what kind of answer was expected. The examiners seem to have interpreted the misunderstanding as stupidity or ignorance. Their failure to rephrase the question was then, probably wrongly, interpreted as malicious. From anecdotes like this one it is easy to see why Asian doctors may be at a disadvantage in viva voce examinations; whether this implies inadequacy on the part of the Asian doctors or cultural bias in the examinations is a difficult question to resolve.

Whether or not they think that biasses occur, many doctors, both British and overseas-qualified, think that doctors from overseas are at a disadvantage in oral examinations because their habits of thought and way of presenting their ideas are very different from what is expected in this country. The general view is that what is expected outside the UK is the general treatment of a theme or subject, giving the opportunity for a display of book learning, whereas what is expected by the Royal College is a succinct treatment of a clinical problem, marshalling of the relevant facts alone, and the logical deduction of a solution. Most overseas doctors concede that the British approach is superior, but think that it takes non-British doctors some time to adapt to its demands. Training activities such as case conferences and journal clubs may be particularly important in helping them to make this adaptation. Certainly, overseas doctors are unlikely to be able to learn a new style of presentation, and to some extent, new habits of thought, without specific practice of some kind.

Social and other problems

The preceding discussion has not been balanced, in that it has concentrated on those overseas doctors who feel resentment about some aspects of their experience in the UK. Those who do not appear to feel any such resentment account for about one-half of those informally interviewed; they tend to be more junior doctors with shorter experience in this country. Among them it is very rare to find doctors who dismiss as illusory the complaints made by others: usually these doctors have simply not been touched by the difficulties that cause resentment in others. There is, in addition, a small group of doctors (much smaller than might appear from the survey) who are acutely conscious of difficulties arising from unequal treatment, but who will not blame the system or individuals in it for treating them in this way.

> 'I have had difficulties in getting jobs because consultants prefer the local lads. Discrimination is natural, it is human nature, we do not complain about it. I could tell you about a case where a job was given to a Liverpool-qualified man who had no membership in preference to an overseas-qualified doctor who had membership. We would do the same in our country. There is discrimination in Pakistan against people from other cities or from other areas.'

But not many overseas doctors go out of their way to excuse the medical establishment for not giving them a fair chance. It is far more common for junior doctors to feel no resentment because the issues have not touched them personally. These junior overseas doctors do not feel rejected by British doctors, but they are usually extremely isolated. Since they have come to the UK temporarily for training, they usually make no effort to get to know the country or the people in it, and attempts to make friends seem particularly valueless to them because they have to move to new jobs and new towns at such short intervals. Ordinary immigrants from India, Pakistan or Africa go to live in areas where many people belonging to their own national, linguistic or religious group are already living. Doctors cannot do this. They nearly always find themselves in areas where there is nobody belonging to their own group, whom they could get to know. Even where there are such people, they tend to be uneducated and working-class, and the barriers of education and class are more important than the ethnic affinity. Asian doctors feel that they have no means of making acquaintances in this country except through the hospitals where they work, and the number of relationships with English doctors that carry over to the home and family are very few. Asian doctors who are unmarried or without their wives or husbands tend to feel extremely isolated, and the wives of those who are married also tend to be very lonely.

A further source of difficulty, and in some cases resentment, among overseas doctors is their relations with administrative staff at the hospital. At more than one of the hospitals that we visited the administrative staff were thought to be racially prejudiced and to show it in the way that they dealt with Asian doctors : one doctor said 'The administrative staff treat us like dirt.' Friction was most likely to arise over accommodation provided by the hospital, with complaints on the one side that requests for repairs and replacements were ignored and on the other that unreasonable demands were made. However, what seemed to be important was not that accommodation was a substantive issue but that the Asian doctors were made to feel uncomfortable whenever they came into contact with administrative staff.

Attitudes of British consultants

A majority of the British consultants whom we informally interviewed were either well-disposed towards overseas doctors, or at least not hostile to them, and where they put forward criticisms this was in a moderate, reasonable and generally constructive spirit. It is, of course, possible that there was some self-selection in the sampling of consultants, leading to an under-representation of those who are hostile to overseas doctors. Our interview with four members of a district management team, if it is a reliable indicator, suggests that this is so. All four agreed that there was considerable prejudice on the part of some consultants against coloured applicants, which went well beyond any ideas about British qualifications being better, or British-qualified doctors having better understanding of the patients, or the fact that an applicant who qualified at a particular medical school might already be known to them. The four varied in the extent to which they felt such prejudice was conscious or overt. Dr. Jones thought that in only one of the many interview panels that he had sat on was there clear intention to discriminate solely on racial grounds; he had refused to go along with this, and the coloured applicant had got the job. Mr. Jamieson and Dr. Baker felt that consultants 'often' took pride in keeping their departments white, or — even more — in getting them white when they had been staffed by overseas doctors. They stated unequivocally that some consultants went down lists of candidates for posts, looked at the names, and then said 'There are only two we can shortlist', meaning that there were only two whites.

Of the two British consultants that we encountered who were hostile to overseas doctors the first was a surgeon in a district general hospital, and also the clinical tutor there. The contrast between Dr. Hastie's forceful extrovert temperament and the shy diffidence of most of the Asian doctors in the hospital was very striking. At the heart of Dr. Hastie's attitude towards overseas doctors was an upper middle-class English exclusiveness: 'You get many overseas applicants for surgical posts, but you tend to appoint the British chap because inevitably you prefer your own kind of person. It's an awful thing to have to say, but when it comes to a

g

crisis you can't be sure that you can rely on an overseas chap, you don't know how he will react.'

Nearly everything that Dr. Hastie said sprang from this basic attitude and was intended to explain why overseas doctors were unsatisfactory, why it was better to avoid employing them if at all possible, and why it was scandalous that the influx of overseas doctors into the country had not been stopped or reduced years ago. A number of specific points were made. Dr. Hastie thought that the language problem was serious; he had himself a language difficulty when practising abroad. He also considered that, because of the language problem, overseas doctors could not sensibly be examined within the same framework as British doctors. It surprised him that doctors with poor English passed the membership and fellowship examinations, and it made him wonder whether the standards were being varied.

Dr. Hastie thought that it was difficult to help overseas doctors to learn, partly because of the language problem, and partly because they would not attend the seminars and discussion groups that were organised. (In fact, most of the seminars and discussion groups for doctors inside the hospital were organised by other consultants, and were attended by overseas doctors, most of whom were not even aware that Dr. Hastie had a special responsibility in this field.)

Another difficulty that Dr. Hastie saw in employing overseas doctors was that many of them intended to go back to the home country shortly, and the hospital did not want to start training a doctor who would then go away. Although the actual appointment might be for only a year, it was often 'expected' that the doctor would stay longer and move up to the next grade. In this way Dr. Hastie justified rejecting applicants who said they would return home within the next few years. Furthermore, he had found that overseas applicants would often say that they intended to stay when they actually meant to leave, and he used this as a justification for turning down overseas applicants in all circumstances: that is, he argued that *you could never be sure* whether they would stay for as long as you expected them to.

While rejecting overseas applicants because they were likely to return home, Dr. Hastie also thought that many of them 'are utterly mad to stay'. Thus, Dr. Hastie criticised overseas doctors both for staying in the UK and for meaning to go away. Presumably what he meant was that those who were incompetent should go home, while those who were competent should stay to commit themselves to permanent or at least lengthy careers in this country.

Dr. Hastie did think that overseas doctors performed a useful function by filling junior posts for which the supply of British graduates was inadequate. The way that he put it was 'In surgery we need a lot of junior pairs of hands.' At the same time he conceded that 'We need to find a way of using overseas doctors that is satisfactory to them.' He did not see that using overseas doctors as 'junior pairs of hands' was precisely what was *not* 'satisfactory to them'.

A second British consultant whose views were definitely hostile to overseas doctors was Dr. Lodge, who was in charge of the anaesthetics department serving a group of hospitals. He was a consultant (of the kind described by the district management team) who took pride in turning a department consisting mainly of overseas-qualified doctors into one that is all-white.[6] Up to two years ago all of the twelve junior doctors in his department had been Asians, whereas now all but one were white and British-qualified. The change had been brought about as a matter of conscious policy by Dr. Lodge, and must have involved unlawful discrimination. Dr. Lodge was highly satisfied with the results of the change. The juniors now passed membership and fellowship examinations more quickly and with less effort on the part of the senior doctors. Furthermore, the department was happier and more easily run, because staff relations were better and the British doctors were more reliable, punctual, competent and 'honourable'.

Dr. Lodge thought that the Asian junior doctors had been slow to learn because their basic medical training was very substantially inferior. He thought there was no problem with Asians who had been through British medical schools. But he also thought that Asians were reluctant to make an effort and took too little advantage of the opportunities that were offered to them. For all of these reasons it was an effort to get them through their examinations.

Unlike Dr. Hastie, Dr. Lodge did not think that the language problem was important: 'We have had no real language problems, all of our overseas graduates have been competent as far as English is concerned'. But overseas graduates were slower to learn, especially to pick up the practical aspects of the specialty, and this was because their basic training was inferior.

However, Dr. Lodge's antagonism to Asians seemed to be related more to their general attitudes and behaviour than to their competence. 'As individuals it is fair to say that their sense of values and priorities is quite different.' What Dr. Lodge meant by this was that Asians are unreliable, devious, even dishonourable. They fail to turn up for interviews, they do not accept jobs on the spot when they are offered to them after the interview, they accept an appointment but then withdraw two days before they are due to start work, they start to look for another job on the first day in the present one, they give one month's notice when doing what is considered to be a two-year registrar job, they take sick leave unnecessarily and are then seen at the Test Match, they cancel patients for operations for minimal medical reasons, they try to take a disproportionate amount of leave, they stay away on sick notes signed by their doctor-spouses. Altogether 'I regret that a high proportion of those from

---

6 This consultant was not known to the district management team, which covered a different area.

India, Pakistan and Bangladesh were different from what we normally expect in medical graduates.'

We cannot say how common views like Dr. Hastie's and Dr. Lodge's are among British consultants; our guess is that they are neither rare nor very common. The destructiveness of these views, and the hostility that goes with them, are the complement to the frustration, resentment and bitterness felt by some overseas doctors.

X Conclusions

Our task in this concluding chapter is to review the relationship between overseas doctors and the National Health Service both from the perspective of overseas doctors and from the perspective of the NHS, to consider whether this is a relationship in which overseas doctors tend to be exploited, and whether there are policies which would prevent any such exploitation while also, if at all possible, improving training programmes, methods of organisation and standards of care in the NHS. We shall begin by summarising the main findings contained in the body of the report.

Summary of the findings

Background. Thirty-one per cent of doctors in the National Health Service in England were born outside the United Kingdom, and a rather smaller proportion (25 per cent) first qualified overseas. Doctors come from a wide range of areas of which the most important are the Indian sub-continent (17 per cent, by country of qualification), Arab countries and Iran (3 per cent) and white anglophone countries (2 per cent). A higher proportion of hospital doctors than of GPs are overseas-qualified (32 per cent compared with 14 per cent). The great majority of overseas-qualified doctors are assessed by interviewers as 'coloured' or 'black' (86 per cent), but 'white anglophones' are an interesting and important group for this study. Overseas-qualified doctors are concentrated within a middle age range: 30-44 years in the case of hospital doctors and 35-54 years in the case of GPs. This is because of the pattern of migration and re-emigration. The balance of the sexes is the same among British and among overseas-qualified doctors. There are substantial proportions of overseas-qualified hospital doctors in every English region of the NHS, and although there are some regional variations in this respect these are not generally very striking. On the other hand, there has been a strong tendency for overseas-qualified GPs to settle in conurbation areas coinciding with the centres of Asian communities. Overseas-qualified doctors are very strongly concentrated within the junior grades of the hospital service: without them it would be impossible to maintain the present ratio of two junior doctors to every one consultant. They are also concentrated within 'shortage' specialties such as geriatrics, psychiatry and anaesthetics, but are under represented in popular specialties such as general medicine and general surgery. Not surprisingly, British-qualified hospital doctors, who tend to be older and more senior, are also more likely than overseas-qualified hospital doctors to have the principal postgraduate qualification, membership or fellowship of a Royal College. However, overseas-qualified GPs tend to have a Higher Postgraduate Qualification in a specialty other than general practice because most of them set out with a hospital career in mind.

Command of English. Thirteen per cent of overseas-qualified doctors are native English speakers in the fullest sense, that is they spoke English, and only English, at home as children; a further 17 per cent spoke English together with another language or languages at this stage. Thus, 70 per cent of overseas doctors are not native English speakers, although most of these were taught in English at medical college, and many were taught in English at school. An objective test of command of English was devised, and was completed by 95 per cent of doctors interviewed. This test, which concentrated on styles of English relevant to a doctor practising in England, was found to have a high reliability, and among indications that the test was valid were the strong relationships between test scores and interviewers' assessments of the informants' English (recorded before the test was administered) and the informants' linguistic background. Among overseas-qualified doctors, 13 per cent scored 14 or less out of 29 on this test, and these doctors certainly have a substantial linguistic handicap. A further 18 per cent scored between 15 and 18, and these probably have a significant linguistic handicap, whereas those scoring 19 or more probably do not. Thus, at least 13 per cent and possibly as many as one-third of overseas doctors have a significant linguistic handicap. The English of overseas doctors tends to improve rapidly as they stay in the UK; few of those who have been in this country for three years or more have a significant handicap. There is also a strong relationship between command of English and seniority within the hospital service. There is no significant language problem among senior registrars and above, or among GPs.

The migration. About one-half of overseas-born doctors came to the UK in the 1970s, about one-quarter in the 1960s and about one-quarter before 1960. At the time of the migration, doctors were typically aged 25-30, though a significant proportion migrated at a later age than this. Among those who were born and first qualified overseas, three-quarters completed two or more years' practice in the country of origin before coming to the UK. About one-half of the migrants were already married when they came to this country, and most of these were either accompanied by their wives or husbands, or were joined by them later, usually within one year. It was more common for migrants to be separated from their children for a time, but only 6 per cent of migrants were separated from a child or children at the time of the interview. A substantial proportion of migrants who are now married (17 per cent of the overseas-qualified not including white anglophones) are married to a British person, and this represents more than one-half of those who have married since coming to the UK and who therefore had the opportunity to marry a British person. These doctors now have close links with this country and are, therefore, less likely to return to their countries of origin. Only 28 per cent of adult migrants obtained information from an official British body about training and career opportunities before coming to this country. Three-quarters of migrants came first and looked for a job when they got here. Among these are 46 per cent who had found a medical job (not necessarily the kind they ideally wanted) within eight weeks and 25 per cent who had difficulties leading, in a substantial minority of cases, to a lengthy period of unemployment.

Reasons for migrating. The great majority (85 per cent) of overseas doctors who migrated as adults came to the UK with the specific aim of obtaining further medical experience, training or qualifications, although this applies rather less strongly to doctors from white anglophone countries than to the rest. Thus, most overseas doctors did not come to the UK to settle, but to complete a stage in their medical training and careers.

Migrants' expectations compared with their experience. Over one half of the migrants (58 per cent) were disappointed in some way with the experience of studying and working in this country; complaints mostly relate to lack of opportunity to get suitable jobs and a lack of time or opportunity for study and training. White anglophones are much less likely to have complaints of this kind than other migrants. Hospital doctors in geriatric posts are especially likely to have a disappointment to express, and specifically to complain about the difficulty of getting a suitable job. In fact, these particular difficulties are mentioned four times as often by those in geriatrics as by those in other specialties. While over one half of the migrants had some disappointment to express, a similar proportion (55 per cent) had found something about studying or working in this country better than they expected. When specifically asked about opportunities for postgraduate medical training in the UK, one-third of migrants said they were disappointed with them (while 56 per cent were pleased). Those who qualified in the UK or a white anglophone country are about half as likely to have been disappointed in their expectations in this respect as those who qualified elsewhere, which suggests that difficulties in gaining access to postgraduate training are greatest for groups which are culturally and racially most distinct from British doctors, and whose basic qualifications are least likely to be considered equivalent to British ones.

Intended and actual length of stay. At the time when they came to the UK, the great majority of migrants intended to stay for a few years only, typically for three to five years. Most of them have either stayed for substantially longer than they meant to or have so far been in the UK for only a short time. A substantial proportion of those who have stayed for longer than they intended have done so because they have not attained their educational, training or career objectives (37 per cent), and a smaller proportion because of the attractions of jobs, careers or more generally life in this country (26 per cent). Marriage and family circumstances are also important reasons for staying. From these findings it seems that migrants who have difficulties in achieving their objectives quickly are more likely to stay for more than a few years than migrants who have few difficulties. This means that among the stock of migrants in the UK at any one time there may be a relatively high proportion who have encountered difficulties, whereas among the flow of migrants coming to the UK over a period, this proportion may be smaller. The present survey, therefore, which is of the stock rather than the flow of doctors, will tend, if anything, to emphasise the difficulties encountered by migrants.

Migrants' aims and achievements. Migrants typically, though not universally, came to the UK intending to pass the membership or fellowship examination of one of the Royal Colleges within a few years, and then to return to the country of origin. Of those who had this typical plan and who have been in this country for nine years or more, less than half (46 per cent) have obtained membership or fellowship, while a further 8 per cent have obtained Part 1 only. Of those having the typical plan and who have been in the UK for five to eight years, 35 per cent have membership or fellowship, and a further 15 per cent have Part 1 only. Thus, upwards of half of migrants who have been in this country for nine years or more have failed in their own terms. Because successful migrants are probably more likely to leave within a short period, it is probable that less than half of all migrants who come to the UK over a defined period are destined to fail. Nevertheless, the proportion who fail in their own terms is a substantial one.

Choice of career. The great majority of overseas-qualified doctors (89 per cent) originally hoped to become specialists, compared with a much smaller proportion of the British-qualified (42 per cent). British-qualified doctors, therefore, comprise a broad spectrum, whereas overseas-qualified doctors are a self-selected group consisting mainly of those who hoped to pursue a career at a high level as specialists and who were prepared to go abroad to gain the necessary training. Doctors from white anglophone countries are like British-qualified doctors in this respect. General practitioners can roughly be divided into those who originally intended to become GPs, and those who originally intended to become specialists but switched to general practice perhaps after failing to make the expected progress in the hospital service. Among British-qualified GPs, those who made a later decision to pursue this career account for 24 per cent of the total, whereas among overseas-qualified GPs (excluding white anglophones), they are the great majority (78 per cent). Some of these late and very late entrants to general practice have chosen the career reluctantly after failing to progress within the hospital service in the UK. Others have decided to remain here (for example because they have married a British person) and have subsequently decided that within the British context they prefer a career in general practice, whereas they would have pursued a specialist career if they had returned to the country of origin. In either case, because overseas-qualifed GPs are mostly late or very late entrants to general practice, they tend to have higher postgraduate qualifications than British-qualified GPs.

Choice of specialty. From comparing original specialty preferences with the actual specialty distribution, we find that overseas-qualified doctors tend to work in the less popular specialties and that they tend to have been channelled into specialties which they did not themselves prefer. These less popular specialties are also, broadly speaking, the shortage specialties, as defined by the DHSS.

Expectations and achievements of British and overseas-qualified doctors compared. We have compared the aims and expectations of migrants with their actual experience and achievements, but we can now add to this an external comparison with British-qualified doctors. All doctors were asked whether, in terms of further study and examinations, they had progressed as fast as they originally expected to, and if not, what had caused their progress to be slower than expected. Twenty per cent of British-qualified doctors, 27 per cent of white anglophones and 55 per cent of other overseas-qualified doctors said they had progressed slower than they expected, which shows that the overseas-qualified (apart from white anglophones) are substantially more likely than the British-qualified to be disappointed with their progress. A lack of opportunity to get good training jobs and a lack of time for study are the reasons most often given for slow progress. Even among those who have now obtained membership or fellowship, the difference between the British and overseas-qualified remains; this shows that it does not arise simply because those who are successful among the overseas-qualified tend to return home. Because overseas-qualified doctors are a self-selected group, a relatively high proportion of them expected to pass the membership or fellowship examinations within ten years of graduating. Among those who had this expectation and who graduated at least ten years ago, a higher proportion of the British-qualified than of the overseas-qualified have achieved their original objective (52 per cent compared with 38 per cent). Among those who graduated less than ten years ago the difference is greater, showing that the overseas-qualified are particularly unlikely to pass the membership or fellowship examinations quickly.

Of course, since three-quarters of migrants obtained no information about study and careers in the UK from an official body before they came, it may be that their expectations were, in some cases, unrealistic.

Transition from the country of origin to the UK. Overseas doctors tend to lose time and seniority when they move from the country of origin to the UK. For example, among those who last worked as registrars abroad (the largest group, accounting for 31 per cent of migrants), only 13 per cent started at the same grade in the UK. Less than 0.5 per cent moved up to a higher grade, 68 per cent slipped back to senior house officer and 10 per cent slipped back to house officer. Overall, two thirds of migrants start at senior house officer level and they tend to start at this level regardless of their previous experience abroad. In terms of time, overseas doctors seem to lose about 30 months on coming to the UK. For example, overseas-qualified doctors who start at senior house officer level in this country have, on average, worked previously for 53 months abroad, whereas British-qualified doctors work, on average, for 22 months before reaching senior house officer level.

Career progress once in the UK. Overseas doctors do not generally retrieve the time that they lose at the time of the migration. If we consider the total time from passing the MB examinations to the date of our interview for this report, we find that among the overseas-qualified, those who have progressed to registrar or senior registrar are still more than 30 months behind their British-qualified counterparts, while those who are still at senior house officer level tend to have fallen further behind. It seems that there is a sub-group of overseas doctors who, having started in the UK usually at senior house officer level, have great difficulty in progressing to a higher grade. Analysis of each of the stages of the career progress separately confirms that among overseas-qualified doctors who do progress from one grade to another the rate of progress is similar to that of British-qualified doctors or only slightly slower, but there is also a group of overseas-qualified doctors who have not progressed. Thus, British-qualified senior house officers have, on average, been senior house officers for 16 months, whereas for overseas-qualified senior house officers the comparable figure is 31 months (counting time in this country only), or almost twice as long.

Seniority and qualifications related to age. Overseas-qualified doctors tend to be in more junior jobs than the British-qualified partly because they tend, on balance, to be younger, but when age is controlled, radical differences in seniority remain. For example, among British-qualified hospital doctors aged 35 to 44, 71 per cent are consultants, compared with only 16 per cent of overseas-qualified doctors in this age group. The lower level of postgraduate qualifications among overseas doctors can be seen as both a cause and a consequence of their relative failure to progress. When we compare British and overseas-qualified hospital doctors within the same age groups according to the highest postgraduate medical qualifications that they possess, we still find substantial differences. Among those aged 30-34 it is not, perhaps, surprising to find that a far higher proportion (74 per cent) of the British-qualified than of the overseas-qualified (19 per cent) have obtained membership or fellowship, since at this stage many of the overseas doctors have been in this country for a comparatively short time. But the differences remain large for the later age groups; thus, among those aged 35-44, 81 per cent of British-qualified hospital doctors have membership or fellowship compared with 43 per cent of the overseas qualified, and although the differences are reduced for later age groups, they remain substantial. A large proportion of overseas-qualified doctors who have stayed in the hospital service in the UK beyond the age of about 40 have never achieved the qualification for which most of them came, and among those who have stayed into late middle age, the great majority are failures in this respect. Many others may have succeeded and returned to the country of origin, but among those who have stayed the failure rate is high.

Seniority related to qualifications. The difference in level of qualifications is related to the difference in seniority; but overseas-qualified doctors are substantially more junior than British doctors with equivalent qualifications. For example, 68 per cent of British-qualified hospital doctors with membership or fellowship are consultants, compared with 28 per cent of overseas doctors with the same postgraduate qualification.

Seniority related to language test score. The difference between British and overseas-qualified doctors in seniority may partly be accounted for by a difference in command of English, although it is difficult to estimate the separate effect of language test score as distinct from other factors to which it is related such as age, length of time spent in the UK and qualifications held.

Seniority compared, with three variables controlled. We have found that overseas doctors are more junior than British doctors partly because they are younger, partly because of imperfect English, and partly because they are less well-qualified. Do these three factors jointly explain the difference in seniority? In order to find out we compared British and overseas-qualified doctors in the age group 28-54 years, who had passed the membership or fellowship examinations, and who scored 21 or more on the language test. The two groups were weighted so that their age profiles were exactly the same. With the three factors controlled in this way, the British-qualified were still twice as likely to be consultants as the overseas-qualified. This finally demonstrates that there is a strong tendency for overseas-qualified doctors whose English is at least adequate to have made less progress in their careers than British doctors of the same age and with comparable qualifications.

Type of registration and career progress. At the time of the survey, 37 per cent of overseas-qualified hospital doctors had been granted not full but only temporary registration; a further 8 per cent were temporarily registered initially, but have since acquired full registration. Although temporarily registered doctors have qualifications that are not recognised for the purpose of full registration, they do often become senior in the hospital service; 16 per cent of overseas-qualified senior registrars and medical assistants and 10 per cent of overseas-qualified consultant are temporarily registered. Further, one-third of overseas-qualified consultants were temporarily registered in their first post in the UK, presumably because their primary qualification was not recognised. Thus, temporarily registered doctors, while they are given second-class status, may often be doing the most responsible jobs. They are not, of course, allowed to work as GPs. There is no evidence that the relatively slow career progress of overseas-qualified doctors is confined to the temporarily registered. On the contrary, doctors who have ever been temporarily registered seem, if anything, to have progressed more quickly than overseas doctors who have always had full (or provisional) registration.

Jobs in teaching districts. The strong tendency for overseas-qualified hospital doctors to be working in non-teaching districts could help to account for their tendency to progress slowly. Only 19 per cent of overseas-qualified hospital doctors (excluding white anglophones) are working in a teaching district or London postgraduate hospital, compared with 45 per cent of British-qualified hospital doctors and a similar proportion of white anglophones (47 per cent). This concentration in non-teaching districts is associated to some extent with inadequate English, but not with any other factor. Nevertheless, even among overseas doctors with good English, penetration into the teaching districts was comparatively low.

Summary of career progress. These findings show that the tendency for overseas doctors to be more dissatisfied with their progress than British doctors is justified by the facts. However, the kind of analysis that we have carried out concentrates on the differences between the two groups. To balance this, it should be remembered that nearly half of overseas doctors have progressed as fast as they expected (compared with three-quarters of British doctors), and that in spite of a tendency for overseas doctors to progress more slowly than comparable British doctors, many do achieve their objectives and progress at similar rates to comparable British doctors. Also, there is some evidence that the more successful overseas doctors tend to return quickly to their countries of origin, and if this is so, any survey of the stock of overseas doctors must be biassed, to some extent, towards those who have been less successful and who are more likely to stay. This is, of course, not so much a bias as a fact about the stock of overseas doctors in the NHS, which may contain a disproportionately high number of the relatively unsuccessful. It is an important finding for the British health services that among those overseas doctors who have remained in the UK for a long period or permanently there is a high proportion who have failed to achieve their training objectives.

Present experience of hospital doctors. From factual and attitudinal questions about the experience of hospital doctors in their present jobs, we found few differences between the British and overseas-qualified.

However, some aspects of training are extremely difficult to assess from survey questions, for example the benefit gained from day-to-day contact with the consultant. As to the attitudinal questions, there are psychological reasons why ratings of the present job always tend to be high, whereas previous jobs are more likely to be criticised. The findings do not, therefore, conclusively establish that the present experience of British and overseas hospital doctors is in fact comparable.

The ethnic and language dimensions in hospital practice. A larger proportion of British-qualified junior doctors (94 per cent) than of the overseas-qualified (86 per cent) have British consultants, which may suggest that there is some tendency for British consultants to prefer British juniors. A substantial minority of doctors (about one-third) think there is little social contact between different ethnic groups in the hospital outside the wards; this view is more common among British than among overseas doctors. One-third of British hospital doctors, but only 10 per cent of the overseas-qualified (excluding white anglophones) think that there are difficulties or shortcomings in working relationships between coloured and white doctors in the hospital. The difficulties mentioned by British doctors were either to do with communication, language or culture, or simply amounted to criticisms of the standards, competence or dedication of overseas doctors. A substantial proportion of British doctors think that the inadequate English of overseas doctors and of patients belonging to minority groups leads to problems in communication. Few overseas doctors think that they have language difficulties of any kind, and where they do think they have difficulties, they are thinking of the inadequacy of other people's English and not of their own. Even overseas doctors who scored very low on the language test very seldom believe that they have difficulties in communication either with other doctors or with patients because of their own inadequate English. This suggests that overseas doctors do tend to underestimate their own language difficulties, or perhaps to be unaware of them. It is a fairly common view among hospital doctors that some patients prefer not to be treated by a coloured doctor, but British doctors emphasise this kind of patient resistance more than overseas doctors do.

Intention to remain in the UK or leave. Just over half (58 per cent) of overseas-qualified hospital doctors in England at the time of the survey said that they intended to leave the country in the foreseeable future, generally within two or three years. Most of those who intend to leave intend to return to the country of origin. Among those who came recently a majority intend to leave again in the future, whereas among those who came some years ago a majority intend to stay. This implies that a majority of the inflow of migrants intend to leave again and actually do so, and in detail the figures suggest that the commonest actual length of stay is between six and ten years (which is much longer than the commonest intended length of stay). Overseas-qualified doctors most commonly intend to leave after reaching registrar or senior registrar level, and they do actually tend to leave at these points. Thus, overseas doctors at the junior grades (registrar and below) are broadly speaking a floating population, whereas those at the more senior grades (senior registrar and above) are mostly permanently settled in the UK.

Present experience of GPs. British-qualified GPs are more likely than overseas-qualified GPs to say that they find problems or difficulties in practising as a GP in England: their complaints relate mainly to 'the system', pay and hours of work. Most GPs are fully reconciled to a career in general practice if they did not choose it in the first place, and in support of their position they argue that general practice offers strong positive advantages over a specialist career. However, a proportion of late entrants still feel that their career is a second best, or that they are out of place in general practice. Because there are far more late entrants among the overseas-qualified, there are also substantially more who see themselves as misfits than among the British-qualified. At a time when there is a movement towards larger group practices which is officially encouraged there is a marked tendency for overseas-qualified GPs to belong to the smaller, one or two-person practices which are generally less desirable and popular. This contrast is particularly strong when we take into account the fact that most overseas doctors entered general practice in the UK recently when small practices were already on the decrease. There is a tendency towards 'racial polarisation' in general practice, that is, a general tendency for coloured doctors, regardless of the particular ethnic group, to cluster together in the same practices. There is no tendency for doctors from white anglophone countries to be grouped with other (coloured) overseas doctors. As far as we can tell within the limitations of a survey method, British-qualified and overseas-qualified GPs handle, on average, about the same total volume of work, but overseas-qualified GPs claim that they work longer hours in handling it. The overseas-qualified are more likely than the British-qualified to use deputising services, largely because they tend to have practices in conurbation and other urban areas where these services are available. The great majority of overseas-qualified GPs have now settled permanently in UK; only 11 per cent expect to leave in the foreseeable future.

Attitudes towards Asian doctors. A majority (60 per cent) of British-qualified doctors say that the average level of competence is lower among Asian than among white British doctors, and 51 per cent say that there is, among Asians, a higher proportion who are below a minimum acceptable standard. The only group of doctors who seldom agree with these views are Asian doctors themselves. Other overseas-qualified doctors often subscribe to these anti-Asian views, though less often than the British-qualified. These views are so prevalent and so forthrightly expressed that they almost certainly influence selection committees.

Selection procedures. The great majority of doctors, whether British or overseas-qualified, think that a coloured, overseas-qualified applicant will have a poorer chance than a white, British-qualified applicant with comparable qualifications and experience when applying for the same hospital job. Thus, it is generally agreed among doctors that overseas applicants do not receive equal treatment. However, this unequal treatment is interpreted as ethnic or racial discrimination by only 18 per cent of the British-qualified, 28 per cent of white anglophones and 18 per cent of other overseas-qualified doctors. The usual interpretation among British-qualified doctors is that selection committees rightly believe that overseas qualifications are inferior or that the overseas doctor is less likely to be competent to practise in the UK. The usual interpretation among the overseas-qualified is that these same judgements are made wrongly. Of course, rejection of overseas applicants on these grounds might in law amount to ethnic or racial discrimination, but most doctors do not see it that way. One-fifth of coloured doctors claim that they have personally experienced discrimination when applying for a hospital job. In a wider context, it is usual for modest claims of personal experience of discrimination such as these, to be accompanied by much more widespread actual discrimination than the claims would suggest. Overseas-qualified doctors (excluding white anglophones) made on average five times as many applications as British-qualified doctors before finding the present job, whereas white anglophones made about the same number of applications as the British. The very high average for the overseas-qualified arises because two-fifths of them made very large numbers of applications and had exceptional difficulties, compared with only 8 per cent of the British-qualified. More detailed analysis of these findings strongly confirms the opinion held by the great majority of doctors that those whose primary qualifications were obtained overseas are less likely to be selected than those whose primary qualifications are British, when applying for the same hospital jobs, even when the two groups have the same UK higher qualifications.

Informal interviews at nine hospitals showed that graduates of British medical schools are usually able to find a suitable succession of training jobs either at the hospital where they trained or at other hospitals within its 'sphere of influence'. By contrast, doctors from overseas do not have the help of a consultant or institution to smooth their path. More generally, while there might appear to be open competition for all junior posts in hospitals, many such posts are actually reserved for favoured candidates, and British doctors are much more likely than overseas doctors to be favoured in this way. These spheres of influence and informal networks can be regarded as systems for helping junior doctors to put together a suitable training programme without which they might be forced into unsuitable jobs. However, in their present form these systems are bound to work strongly to the disadvantage of any group that does not 'belong'. It is because of these systems that comparatively few overseas doctors find jobs in teaching districts. We have carried out informal interviews at only nine hospitals, which may not be representative. From these interviews we have gained the impression that country of qualification is quite openly used as a criterion of choice by consultants and selection committees, but that doctors who admit a preference for British or white anglophone junior doctors do not usually think they are betraying a prejudice or engaging in acts of ethnic or racial discrimination. Overseas doctors who have exceptional difficulties in finding jobs probably have these difficulties because they do not use informal networks and because they will not abandon their choice of specialty or accept jobs in which training opportunities are poor, and not because they have inferior qualifications, experience or competence. Although we find from the survey that only a minority of overseas doctors accuse selection committees of discriminating on ethnic or racial grounds, there is fairly widespread bitterness and resentment among overseas doctors about their experience of coming to work and train in the UK.

The policy implications

Over the past fifteen to twenty years, medical manpower in the UK has been boosted by the unplanned influx of overseas doctors to compete on the open market for 'training jobs' in the NHS. This inflow has serviced a rapid expansion of the NHS at a time when the supply of home graduates was increasing very little. On one view, this is an exchange of manpower for training and experience which is beneficial to all three interest groups: the NHS, the overseas doctors and the medical systems in their countries of origin. The NHS gains a supply of junior doctors to service its expansion. In addition, since most overseas doctors return to their home countries before becoming consultants, they constitute a constantly refreshed pool of juniors. Because this pool exists, there can be a much larger number of junior doctors in relation to consultants than would otherwise be possible; this allows hospitals to be organised in a way that some consultants prefer. The overseas doctors gain the training, experience and qualifications for which they came to this country. When they return home, the medical systems in the countries of origin, which do not yet have the resources to provide medical training at an advanced level in all the specialties, gain a supply of doctors fully trained in the methods of modern medicine.

This study has shown that the view that the relationship between overseas doctors and the NHS is reciprocally beneficial is too simple. Although there are benefits on both sides, the relationship also has harmful effects both on overseas doctors and on the organisation of the NHS. Taking, first, the perspective of overseas doctors, we find that three-quarters of them came to the UK without first obtaining information from an official body about opportunities here for study and training. A similar proportion, probably the same group, came to this country first and looked for a job when they got here. By and large, therefore, their migration was not planned in conjunction with the British authorities, but happened spontaneously. In these circumstances there could be no guarantee that the migrants' expectations or objectives could be fulfilled. In practice, a large number of the migrants, probably a majority of those who come to the UK, do achieve their training objectives (though not usually within the expected timetable), and do progress at broadly comparable rates to British doctors. However, a substantial proportion do not achieve their training objectives within a reasonable timetable or at all, and are seriously disappointed with their experience in this country and, in many cases, are bitter and resentful. Overseas doctors do objectively tend to have much greater difficulties in finding jobs than British doctors, and it is widely believed by all groups of doctors, at all levels, that the overseas-qualified are not able to compete on equal terms with British doctors on the job market, or thus to gain equal access to good training jobs. Regardless of how this is interpreted — whether as institutionalised discrimination based on racism or as the proper exercise of judgement by selection committees — it is bound to lead to the exploitation of overseas doctors, among whom an important proportion carry out some of the least popular medical work in the health service without obtaining the training for which they came here.

The shortcomings of the relationship from the point of view of the NHS, though perhaps less obvious, are also serious. The wrong specialties are manned by overseas doctors. Psychiatry and geriatrics in which overseas doctors are especially concentrated are precisely the specialties in which a lack of English and of Englishness are a real handicap to a doctor practising in this country. Within the present medical career and management structure, junior doctors carry out much of the medical work in hospitals, and the amount and quality of supervision is variable. This system may work well where the junior doctors are known quantities, are products of the local medical school, and belong to the local culture. It probably works less well where they are often new arrivals from a foreign country whose medical training is unfamiliar to the consultant. It is a serious difficulty that not all overseas doctors succeed in completing their training programmes, and especially that failure to achieve training objectives is one important reason why doctors stay on in this country. This means that the countries of origin tend to receive back the successful doctors (who may also be more able) while the NHS tends to retain the unsuccessful ones (who may be less able). As an illustration of this pattern, we find that among the older age groups a high proportion of overseas-qualified doctors in the hospital service have not passed the membership or fellowship examinations of the Royal Colleges.

However, the most seriously harmful effect for the NHS is that the use of a transitory population of overseas doctors to do junior jobs allows an artificial structure to develop in which two-thirds of hospital doctors are juniors. In a self-sufficient system these ratios would have to be roughly reversed (about one-third juniors to two-thirds consultants). There are powerful reasons for thinking that the artificial structure is not desirable.

First and foremost, only consultants are fully trained and considered to have all the skills and accomplishments required to practise a specialty: yet a large part of the treatment will actually be carried out by junior doctors, if junior doctors predominate in the service. If, instead, most of the treatment were actually carried out by consultants this would indisputably raise the standard of the service. (In order to appreciate the force of this argument, it has to be remembered that medicine is largely a personal service. The less accomplished doctor may be under supervision, but he is the one who treats the patient; being less accomplished, he will not do the job as well as his consultant.)

Secondly, a higher ratio of consultants would lead to a more rational method of organising medical work in hospitals. Where juniors are doing the bulk of the medical work they are bound to work frequently without effective supervision. If the proportion of juniors were smaller, then a junior doctor would genuinely be working alongside a consultant much of the time, rather than working independently but to instructions. In many specialties a flat as opposed to a hierarchical structure would probably be better suited to the functional demands of the job.

Thirdly, training would be much more effective if there were a higher proportion of consultants who could, therefore, give more time to each junior.[1]

Output from British medical schools has now begun to increase, and this increased output will, according to DHSS forecasts, lead to a diminishing proportion of overseas doctors in the NHS from the second half of the 1980s onwards. Nevertheless, on all current projections, very substantial numbers of overseas doctors will continue to come to the UK for many years ahead if the NHS is to continue to expand at the modest rate expected. We have argued that the present relationship between overseas doctors and the NHS is seriously defective from the perspective of both parties; since the relationship is bound to continue, it is essential to find policies that will improve it.

Anti-discrimination policies

We have not been able to carry out objective tests which would conclusively establish whether and how far there is ethnic or racial discrimination against overseas doctors, and we have pointed out that there are philosophical and legal difficulties in this context in separating judgements about the worth of qualifications and experience from ethnic or racial bias. Most doctors think that the overseas-qualified, as job applicants, are unequally treated, and we see no reason to contradict this view; in fact, many of the consequences of unequal treatment have been documented and analysed in this study. Whether and in what

---

[1] The cost of changing the ratio of consultants to juniors would have to be considered. Increased salary costs because of a higher average level of seniority among hospital doctors might be offset, to a greater or lesser extent, by a reduction in the total manpower required to deliver a given level and quality of service.

circumstances this unequal treatment amounts either to direct or to indirect discrimination under the 1976 Race Relations Act is a question that will only be resolved as examples of the application of the new law become available. We do, however, consider that full consideration should be given to the applicability of the law in this field.

It is important that the question as to what counts as discrimination should be tackled. It is also important that the workings of selection committees should be directly investigated (as they were not in this study) to establish whether, and how far, discrimination enters into them. These objectives could be achieved by means of a formal investigation by the Commission for Racial Equality, and we suggest that the Commission should consider whether to start a formal investigation after weighing the findings of this report.

While the application of the law in this field certainly cannot be ignored, and while the implementation of the law, if it turns out to be applicable, would have a significant impact, this would not radically alter the situation of overseas doctors. They are bound to be at a disadvantage compared with British doctors in putting together a training programme within the present system even if they are fairly treated on the basis of their qualifications and experience. This is because a young doctor arriving in a foreign country whose language he speaks imperfectly and whose people he does not know, who has no contacts with the local medical schools or medical hierarchy, who does not understand the system of practice and training, who is not familiar with the different hospitals, and knows nothing of the opportunities, facilities and prestige attaching to them, is bound to have an uphill struggle in putting together his own training programme from a succession of jobs for which he has to compete on the open market. While, therefore, the law against racial discrimination has a role to play, we believe that most of the inequities in the present system (from the perspective of overseas doctors) arise from structural factors rather than from individual acts or settled policies of racial discrimination.

The training system and immigration policy
At present British and overseas-qualified doctors have to put together their own training programmes by finding a suitable succession of junior jobs. It is quite possible — in fact easy — for a doctor to fail to do this, so that he takes a successsion of junior jobs which do not individually or collectively provide the training and experience that he requires. Overseas doctors are more vulnerable because they have no British teaching hospital to smooth their path, but British doctors may also have difficulties. There is no general system that ensures, or tries to ensure, that junior doctors receive an appropriate programme of training and experience over, say, a seven-year period.

At the same time, overseas doctors come to this country usually without having arranged a job beforehand, often without having obtained proper information about the opportunities available, in many cases perhaps with false expectations, and hope to find the right jobs in the most popular specialties when they arrive. The relationship between overseas doctors and the NHS can be improved to the benefit of both parties if changes are made in both of these conditions.

The NHS should move towards a system in which all junior hospital jobs (like all senior registrar jobs now) form part of planned training programmes that offer a suitable variety of training and experience over a much longer time span than the present six-month or one-year posts. Training programmes of this kind can be regarded as an extension of the principle of rotating posts. Ultimately, all junior hospital posts, instead of being available on the open market, would be points of rotation within training programmes, which would be organised and administered at regional level within the NHS. These programmes would probably have to be divided into a few sections corresponding to the main phases of a hospital doctor's training. For example, there might be a two-year programme covering the present two years as house officer (pre and post registration), a three to four-year programme, covering the present senior house officer and registrar grades, and a two to three-year programme, corresponding to the present training programme for senior registrars. Each of these training programmes would be organised like a repertoire of rotating posts. Doctors would be allocated to a series of posts in response to their training needs, and in such a way that no individual doctor was given only the best or only the poorest posts. Efforts would be made to co-ordinate teaching activities inside and outside hospitals with the needs of the training programmes.

The first phase of the training programmes, covering the two years as house officer, would be split into a general practice option and a specialist option. The general practice option would be similar to the three-year training programme for GPs that is now being introduced, and would include time in general practice. The specialist option would be two years at house officer level in a variety of posts. Both of these options should be largely or entirely conceived for graduates from British medical schools. The training and experience provided at that stage is not highly specialised, and doctors should be able to gain similar experience in their countries of origin before coming to the UK. There may be a difficulty that some overseas doctors need to have some experience of British medicine before competing for entry to the main phase of the training programme. If this is so, the need could be met by providing a limited number of six-month posts for overseas doctors, who would be eligible for such a post once only. This would be a more suitable way of meeting the difficulty than admitting overseas doctors to the first phase of the training programme, which would probably, in a majority of cases, not be appropriate to their needs.

There is bound to be strong competition for training that leads to consultant status. From the survey, we know that many doctors try to pursue a hospital career, but switch to general practice after failing to make the expected progress (whereas very few switch careers in the opposite direction). Under the current arrangements, competition is more or less continuous, since senior house officer posts generally last for 12 months and registrar posts for 2 years. There is room at the early stages of the career structure for more doctors than can progress to consultant status, even allowing for re-emigration of overseas doctors. Doctors who are not going to reach consultant status are not rejected at the outset, but drop out at some later stage when they finally realise that their progress is too slow.

Within a system of training programmes, competition would not be continuous, but would be focussed at the entry points to the two main phases (that is, the phase after the equivalent of the pre and post registration years as house officer). This has the great advantage that, once he has entered a training programme, the junior doctor is freed from the worry of finding his next job. Within such a system, the methods of regulating entry are, of course, a crucial consideration. A suitable method might be by some form of examination. Although selection would presumably be carried out by the regional health authorities (or by special committees set up by them for the purpose) there would be a case for standardising selection procedures nationally, to some extent, so that efforts could be made to remove cultural bias. At the first main phase of the programme (that is, after the two years as house officer), doctors would be joining the stream for a particular specialty (although there could be arrangements for switching specialties later). Because of the widely differing balances between supply and demand as between the different specialties, entry requirements, while never falling below a minimum acceptable standard, would have to be stiffer for some specialties than for others. It would probably be necessary for applicants to give a second and third choice of specialty in case the competition in their first-choice specialty was too stiff for them.

Overseas doctors should be discouraged from entering the country to work in the NHS unless they have previously gained a place within a training programme. On the one hand, only doctors who could meet the entry requirements of the training programmes would be admitted to the country to work in the NHS. On the other hand, the system would ensure that those accepted for training programmes, and who had been admitted to the country, would receive appropriate training and experience, and migrants would be sure to know what they were coming to, before they came.

British and overseas doctors would compete on an equal footing for places in training programmes. This raises the difficult question of how entry into training programmes would be tied in with entry into the UK. Certainly, it would be essential to make arrangements so that overseas doctors could compete at a number of centres abroad for places in the training programmes; if they had to come to the UK to compete, this

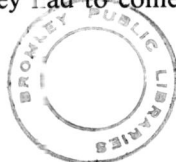

201

would destroy one of the main objectives, which is to encourage people to come only when their place in a training programme is secure. On the other hand, it would not be right to deny entry to doctors unless they had already been accepted on a training programme. Doctors may wish to come to the UK to work in the private sector of medicine or to do research or teaching at a university. Also, as already mentioned, it may be that there should be provision of some six-month junior posts for overseas doctors who need to have some experience of British medicine before competing for entry into a training programme. Finally, if young overseas doctors can support themselves in the UK while preparing to take the examination for entry to a training programme, perhaps they should not be barred from trying to do so.

Probably the best approach is to allow implications for immigration control to flow from the changes in medical training and career structures, rather than vice versa. Doctors would not normally be allowed to enter the country for more than a limited period unless they either had a job to go to or had good prospects of finding one. Under the proposed arrangements, this criterion would still apply. However, if and when all or nearly all junior medical jobs in the NHS are points of rotation within training programmes, overseas doctors will have few prospects of supporting themselves unless they can gain entry to such programmes, and this would affect the view that the immigration authorities would take of applications to enter the UK. In practice, most overseas doctors would have gained entry to a training programme before coming to this country, although there would be no regulation to this effect. Of course, some doctors might come to work in universities or in the private sector, and later try to gain entry to training programmes. This would be quite acceptable, particularly since the numbers entering the system in this way would be fairly small.

So far it has been suggested that overseas doctors should compete on equal terms with British doctors for places on training programmes that have been designed to prepare doctors to be consultants within the British system. To this it may be objected that many overseas doctors do not require such extensive training, or at any rate the same training, as doctors intending to become consultants in the UK. This raises the question as to whether there should be shortened or specialised training programmes designed with the needs of overseas doctors particularly in mind.

This is a question that needs to be seriously considered. It is difficult to say, at present, what overseas doctors would ideally like to get out of coming to train in this country, because their views of what they want are heavily conditioned by what is actually available. We know that a majority of overseas doctors hope to pass the membership or fellowship examinations of a Royal College before returning to the country of origin. However, it may be argued that these qualifications are often, in fact, irrelevant to their subsequent careers, and that if an alternative kind of training were available, leading to a different and more appropriate qualification, then this kind of training and qualification might be very much in demand.

However, the arguments on the other side are fairly strong. As matters stand most overseas doctors stay for substantially more than three years. Within a unitary system of training programmes, the second phase would probably take three or four years and would roughly correspond with the present senior house officer and registrar grades. At the end of this phase, doctors would normally take the membership or fellowship examination. For overseas doctors who wish to come to the UK for training and then return to the country of origin, this phase of the training programme may well be the appropriate solution. Certainly, it does not seem appropriate for those intending to return home to go on to the senior registrar phase. Perhaps entry into this phase should carry with it some explicit commitment to practice in the UK for a period afterwards.

Secondly, there is a serious danger — even a probability — that alternative short programmes would effectively become second-class programmes comprising all the least desirable junior jobs which overseas doctors currently tend to do. This seems a very powerful argument that ought to rule out this option unless standard training programmes can be shown to be totally unsuited to the needs of some overseas doctors whom the NHS wishes to employ.

One reason for suggesting that there ought to be special shortened or watered-down training programmes for overseas doctors is that this would ensure that the majority of overseas doctors would not be in a position to stay in the UK permanently, because they would not have received the 'mainstream' training or passed the examinations normally required of consultants. However, we believe that this reasoning is false, and indeed, the argument can be stood on its head. Overseas doctors who are capable of passing successfully through a training programme should be encouraged to stay in this country. It is in the interest of the NHS, having invested in their training, to retain them as consultants. To the extent that fully-trained overseas doctors do stay in the UK, this will help to change the ratio of juniors to consultants in favour of consultants, and we have already pointed out that such a change can only lead to an improvement in the quality of the service offered by the NHS. Anyone who advocates a system that ensures that most overseas doctors do not stay is making the assumption that their standards will be lower than those of British-trained doctors. But one of the objectives of the training system should be to ensure that this is not the case.

A system of training programmes of the kind that we have discussed would have a number of advantages, some of them affecting the relationship between overseas doctors and the NHS, others of a much more general nature.

First, the system would ensure that junior doctors, once accepted into a training programme, would receive a suitable balance of training and experience in their specialty, or at any rate the best that can be provided with current resources. Thus, junior doctors, whatever their country of qualification, would have much more secure expectation of receiving appropriate training and experience than they do under the present arrangements, where they themselves have to find a series of jobs.

Secondly, unequal treatment as between British and overseas doctors would be eliminated once they had entered a programme, and special efforts could be made to ensure that the criteria used at the initial entry point were fair.

Thirdly, overseas doctors would generally come to the UK with their training programme already arranged, and without false expectations.

Fourthly, the system would be a more efficient method of producing trained doctors than the present one, if within a well planned programme, a higher proportion of the training and experience provided could be useful and relevant. The time taken to produce a consultant might, therefore, be reduced, thus helping to increase the total number of consultants relative to the number of juniors.

Fifthly, pressure would develop to improve the training provided in unsatisfactory junior posts, which would now form rotation points within training programmes, and would immediately be subject to criticism if they provided no training.

Finally, the great majority of doctors accepted into the system, whether from the UK or from overseas, should achieve their training objectives, if the system could be made to work, for doctors would not be accepted unless they showed the necessary potential, and once accepted, they would receive the necessary range of training and experience. It would directly benefit the NHS as well as individual doctors, if there were no longer a group of unsuccessful doctors (mainly from overseas) remaining up to a late age in the hospital service.

The suggestion that the career structure of junior hospital doctors might be reorganised within a system of training programmes is one that emerges out of a study of the special position of overseas doctors, but which has much wider implications. Special study of the medical postgraduate educational system would be required to develop and evaluate this suggestion further. Whatever the exact formulation, it seems that only this kind of policy is capable of changing those aspects of the relationship between overseas doctors and the NHS that work to the disadvantage of both parties, while also helping to achieve other vital objectives.

Appendix A
Additional Tables

List of Additional Tables

A 1 Interviewer's assessment of race or colour, by country of birth.

A 2 Interviewer's assessment of race or colour, by country of first qualification.

A 3 Age and sex, by type of job and country of qualification.

A 4 Proportion of unmarried doctors, by sex and type of job.

A 5 Proportion of hospital doctors born outside the UK and Eire, by Regional Health Authority.

A 6 Proportion of GPs who first qualified outside the UK or Eire, by region (Regional Health Authority).

A 7 Language test: responses to individual items, by country of qualification.

A 8 Language test score, by earliest context in which English was used: overseas-qualified doctors.

A 9 Language test score, by country of first qualification.

A10 Language test score, by grade of post: overseas-qualified hospital doctors.

A11 Year of first coming to the UK, by country of birth: doctors born outside the United Kingdom.

A12 Age on coming to the UK, by country of birth.

A13 Sources of information about medical training or careers in the UK.

A14 Expectations about studying or working in the UK: adult migrants and various subgroups.

A15 Attitudes towards training and experience obtained in the UK: adult migrants and various subgroups.

A16 Salary expectations and experience, by type of post and country of first qualification: adult migrants.

A17 Intended length of stay on coming to the UK, by year of coming: adult migrants.

A18 Actual and intended length of stay in the UK, by year of coming to the UK: adult migrants.

A19 Present grade of adult migrants who expected to reach registrar grade before leaving the UK, by year of coming to the UK.

A20 Present grade of adult migrants who expected to reach senior registrar, medical assistant or consultant grade before leaving, by year of coming to the UK.

A21 Progress in terms of further study and examinations, by country of qualification.

A22 Qualification expectations (within ten years of obtaining MB), by type of job and country of first qualification.

A23 Proportion of hospital doctors working in a teaching district, by country of qualification and grade.

A24 Proportion of hospital doctors in selected specialties who are working in a teaching district, by country of qualification.

A25 Proportion of hospital doctors working in a teaching district, by country of qualification and language test score.

A26 Proportion of hospital doctors working in a teaching district, by country of qualification and highest postgraduate qualification.

A27 Present job type and grade by age: British and overseas-qualified doctors compared.

A28 Highest qualification by age: British and overseas-qualified hospital doctors compared.

A29 Job type and grade, by highest postgraduate qualification: British and overseas-qualified doctors compared.

A30 Grade of hospital doctors, by language test score: British and overseas-qualified doctors compared.

A31 Highest qualification, by language test score: British and overseas-qualified hospital doctors compared.

A32 Total hours spent working or on call in one week: hospital doctors by grade and country of qualification.

A33 Hours spent actually working in one week: hospital doctors by grade and country of qualification.

A34 Hours spent actually working in one week: hospital doctors by specialty.

A35 Number of mornings and afternoons off for study in a four-week period: junior hospital doctors, by grade and country of qualification.

A36 Contact with postgraduate tutor, by country of qualification.

A37 Number of hours spent per week in organised study, by country of qualification.

A38 Country for which hospital doctors intend to leave the UK, by country of qualification.

A39 Reasons for leaving the UK in future: hospital doctors who intend to leave, by country of qualification.

A40 Grade hospital doctors expect to reach before leaving the UK, by country of qualification.

A41 Reasons for preferring to be a hospital doctor: GPs, by country of qualification.

A42 Reasons for preferring to remain a GP, by country of qualification.

A43 Number of doctors in practice, by country of qualification and years in general practice of informant.

A44 Mean number of visits made to patients in an average week: GPs, by country of qualification and age.

A45 Mean number of weekends on call out of every four: GPs, by country of qualification and number of doctors in the practice.

A46 Mean number of weekday nights on call out of every twenty: GPs, by country of qualification and number of doctors in the practice.

A47 Mean hours worked during one week: GPs, by country of qualification and number of doctors in the practice.

A48 Mean hours worked during one week: GPs, by country of qualification and years spent in general practice.

A49 Use of deputising services: GPs, by size of practice.

A50 Number of job applications made before finding the present job: hospital doctors by various factors.

Table A1   Interviewer's assessment of race or colour, by country of birth

Column percentages

	Total	UK/ Eire	Other Europe	White anglo- phone country	Indian sub- cont- inent	Arab country	Other country
				Country of birth:			
White	76	99	83	88	4	16	19
Brown/coloured	20	*	5	10	95	35	43
Black/negroid	1	—	—	2	*	2	17
Other or mixed non-white[1]	3	*	12	1	1	48	21
Base: All informants							
Unweighted	*1,981*	*812*	*127*	*96*	*670*	*133*	*143*
Weighted	*4,490*	*3,119*	*152*	*124*	*752*	*157*	*187*

1 Other types (for example, Japanese characteristics) or mixture of non-white types.

Table A2   Interviewer's assessment of race or colour, by country of first qualification

Column percentages

	Total	UK/ Eire	Not UK/ Eire	White anglo- phone country	Indian sub- cont- inent	Arab country	Other country
				Country of first qualification:			
White	76	97	14	84	1	3	37
Brown/coloured	20	2	74	11	97	37	27
Black/negroid	1	*	2	2	*	2	15
Other or mixed non-white[1]	3	1	10	4	1	58	21
Base: All informants							
Unweighted	*1,981*	*1,016*	*965*	*73*	*664*	*111*	*117*
Weighted	*4,490*	*3,382*	*1,108*	*104*	*748*	*119*	*137*

1 Other types (for example, Japanese characteristics) or mixture of non-white types.

Table A3   Age and sex, by type of job and country of qualification

Column percentages

	General Practitioners (GPs):			Hospital doctors:		
	All GPs	British quali-fied	Over-seas quali-fied	All hospital doctors	British quali-fied	Over-seas quali-fied
Age						
Up to 29 years	4	4	*	29	35	18
30-34 years	14	15	8	22	14	39
35-44 years	28	24	57	23	19	30
45-54 years	32	33	24	13	16	7
55 years and over	22	24	11	13	16	5
Sex						
Male	86	87	82	82	81	84
Female	14	13	18	18	19	16
Base: All informants						
Unweighted	*730*	*477*	*253*	*1,251*	*539*	*712*
Weighted	*1,923*	*1,649*	*274*	*2,567*	*1,733*	*834*

Table A4   Proportion of unmarried doctors, by sex and type of job

Per cent

	Men	Women
Percentage of each of the following groups who are unmarried:		
All doctors	11	37
General practitioners	1	26
Hospital doctors	18	44
British-qualified		
All doctors	9	38
General practitioners	1	28
Hospital doctors	16	45
Overseas-qualified		
All doctors	16	34
General practitioners	3	16
Hospital doctors	21	40

Table A5 Proportion of hospital doctors born outside the UK and Eire, by Regional Health Authority

Regional Health Authority	Per cent
Northern	37
Yorkshire	39
Trent	33
East Anglia	29
NW Thames	32
NE Thames	38
SE Thames	32
SE Thames	32
Wessex	24
Oxford	28
South Western	20
West Midlands	38
Mersey	34
North Western	40
London Postgraduate Teaching Hospitals	24

Source: Hospital Medical Staff — England and Wales, Regional Tables, Department of Health and Social Security, based on the return of 30 September 1977.

Table A6 Proportion of General Practitioners who first qualified outside the UK or Eire, by region (Regional Health Authority)

Region (pairs of RHAs)	Per cent
Northern and Yorkshire	12
Trent and East Anglia	10
NW and NE Thames	27
SW and SE Thames	13
Wessex and South Western	3
Oxford and West Midlands	22
Mersey and North Western	19

Source: PSI survey.

Table A7   Language test: responses to individual items, by country of qualification

Percentage correctly answering each item

	Doctors who first qualified in:		
	UK/Eire (a)	Elsewhere (b)	(a) — (b)[1]
Nouns			
Pink eye	93	89	4
Scurf	99	71	28
Thrush	98	92	6
The change	100	88	12
Acid head[2]	50	22	28
Cissy	88	52	36
Warts	99	89	10
Boil	99	98	1
Ringworm	98	88	10
Adam's apple	100	95	5
Phrases			
Keep your hair on	97	68	29
He is crackers	99	81	18
I am whacked	100	70	30
She had the curse	96	58	38
I am all bunged up	98	62	36
He flew off the handle	96	65	31
He was a bit tight	94	56	38
She was full of beans	98	63	35
His girlfriend was in the club	91	42	49
He could no longer get it up	95	78	17
Verbs with prepositions			
Broken down	97	81	16
Bring him round	96	69	27
Come up against	97	84	13
Getting about	90	72	18
Keep it up	94	77	17
Looking forward to	99	87	12
Makes out that	67	39	28
Put up with	99	85	14
Feeling run down	99	85	14
Takes off famous people	94	31	63

Base: Informants who completed
     the language test

[1] The arithmetic subtraction of the figures in column (b) from column (a) gives an indication of the degree of understanding of overseas-qualified doctors.
[2] Excluded from the full test score.

NB: The wording of the items in this table has been shortened. For the full wording (and multiple choices) see the language test reproduced in Appendix C.

Table A8 Language test score, by earliest context in which English was used: overseas-qualified doctors

Column percentages

	\multicolumn{6}{c}{Spoke/used English:}
	As child at home, only language	As child at home, with other languages	At school and college	At college, not at school	At school, not at college	None of these
0-14	2	8	12	29	20	23
15-18	1	14	19	24	23	16
19-23	15	28	34	35	30	25
24-25	10	19	14	3	7	7
26-27	23	16	10	5	7	11
28-29	48	6	5	3	2	10
Test not done	2	8	6	2	7	8
Base: Overseas-qualified doctors						
Unweighted	*92*	*156*	*560*	*58*	*42*	*57*
Weighted	*149*	*190*	*596*	*66*	*46*	*61*

NB: the horizontal classification in this table is hierarchical.

Table A9 Language test score, by country of first qualification

Column percentages

Language test score	UK/Eire	All overseas	White anglo-phone country	Indian sub-continent	Arab country	Other coun-tries
0-14	—] *	12] 28	—] —	12] 29	18] 46	16] 32
15-18	*]	16]	—]	17]	28]	16]
19-23	1	30	8	34	28	28
24-25	4	13	17	14	12	7
26-27	22	12	21	12	5	12
28-29	68	10	50	6	3	8
Test not done	4	6	4	6	6	13
Base: All informants						
Unweighted	*1,016*	*965*	*73*	*664*	*111*	*117*
Weighted	*3,382*	*1,108*	*104*	*748*	*119*	*137*

Table A10   Language test score, by grade of post: overseas-qualified hospital doctors

Column percentages

	HO/SHO[1]	Registrar	Grade: Senior registrar	Medical assistant	Consultant	Grade not known
0-14	25 ⎤ 50	11 ⎤ 32	— ⎤ 9	3 ⎤ 13	2 ⎤ 7	21 ⎤ 28
15-18	25 ⎦	21 ⎦	9 ⎦	10 ⎦	5 ⎦	7 ⎦
19-23	29	38	26	37	12	52
24-25	9	13	23	13	12	7
26-27	4	10	7	20	31	—
28-29	2	5	25	13	26	3
Test not done	5	3	11	3	13	10

Base: Overseas-qualified hospital doctors

Unweighted	*311*	*233*	*33*	*26*	*85*	*25*
Weighted	*360*	*257*	*57*	*30*	*101*	*29*

1 House officer/Senior house officer

**Table A11   Year of first coming to the UK, by country of birth:
doctors born outside the United Kingdom**

Column percentages

	Total	Conti- nental Europe	Country of birth: White anglo- phone country	Indian sub- conti- nent	Arab country/ Iran	Else- where
Year of first coming to the UK						
Up to 1939	8	33	10	3	8	9
1940-1949	6	21	17	2	5	8
1950-1959	9	12	13	8	4	10
1960-1964	10	2	22	11	5	9
1965-1969	17	6	4	23	9	20
1970-1972	11	6	7	11	19	13
1973-1974	17	6	3	20	29	11
1975-1976	16	10	11	18	19	16
1977-1978	5	3	11	5	3	2
Not stated	1	1	2	—	—	3
Summary						
Up to 1959	23	66	40	13	17	27
1960-1969	27	8	26	34	14	29
1970-1974	28 ⎤ 49	12 ⎤ 25	10 ⎤ 32	21 ⎤ 44	48 ⎤ 70	24 ⎤ 52
1975-1978	21 ⎦	13 ⎦	22 ⎦	23 ⎦	22 ⎦	28 ⎦
Not stated	1	1	2	—	—	3

Base: Doctors born outside the British Isles

Unweighted	*1,169*	*127*	*96*	*670*	*133*	*143*
Weighted	*1,371*	*152*	*124*	*752*	*157*	*187*

Q4 Not counting short visits of less than 6 months, in what month and year did you first come to Britain?

Table A12 Age on coming to the UK by country of birth

Column percentages

	Total	Continental Europe	White anglophone country	Indian subcontinent	Arab country	Elsewhere
			Country of birth:			

Age on coming to the UK

	Total	Continental Europe	White anglophone country	Indian subcontinent	Arab country	Elsewhere
Up to 18 years	16	40	30	5	16	35
19-24 years	7	10	9	6	5	10
25-27 years	26 ⎤49	26 ⎤35	24 ⎤38	30 ⎤58	26 ⎤56	13 ⎤28
28-30 years	23 ⎦	9 ⎦	14 ⎦	28 ⎦	30 ⎦	15 ⎦
31-34 years	16	9	14	19	13	16
35 years or over	9	7	7	11	10	7
Not stated	1	1	2	*	—	3

Base: Doctors born outside the British Isles

	Total	Continental Europe	White anglophone country	Indian subcontinent	Arab country	Elsewhere
Unweighted	*1,169*	*127*	*96*	*670*	*133*	*143*
Weighted	*1,371*	*152*	*124*	*752*	*157*	*187*

Table A13 Sources of information about medical training or careers in the UK

Percentages

	Total	Year of coming to Britain:	
		Up to 1969	1970-1978
British bodies			
General Medical Council	8	3	13
British Medical Association	5	6	4
British Embassy/Consul/High Commission	9	8	10
Department of Health and Social Security	3	*	6
Council for Post Graduate Medical Education	3	4	2
A Royal College	2	3	1
Any of these	**28**	**22**	**32**
Overseas Doctors' Association	*	—	*
Other British bodies	5	6	4
Any British body	**32**	**27**	**35**
Foreign bodies:			
A postgraduate medical association	3	3	4
Social security bodies	*	*	*
Appointments Board of own university or college	3	4	3
Other bodies	4	7	3
Any foreign body	**11**	**13**	**9**
Any British or foreign body	**40**	**37**	**43**
Other doctors:			
Senior colleague/consultant	8	6	10
Professor/teacher	14	16	13
Other local doctors	5	5	6
Visiting doctors from Great Britain	1	1	2
Other students	1	*	1
Any other doctors or students	**28**	**26**	**30**
Friends/relatives:			
In Britain at the time	11	11	10
Who train or had worked in Britain	12	10	13
Who had lived (not trained or worked) in Britain	2	2	3
Friends/relatives unspecified	15	15	14
Any friends/relatives connected with GB[1]	**23**	**20**	**26**
Miscellaneous:			
Journals/magazines/books	8	9	8
Other sources of information	4	5	3
Not stated	7	11	4
Base: Adult migrants			
Unweighted	*1,016*	*437*	*579*
Weighted	*1,160*	*493*	*667*

Q11 From what source or sources did you obtain information about medical training or careers in Britain before you came?

1 Not including 'friends/relatives unspecified'.

Table A14 Expectations about studying or working in the UK:
adult migrants and various subgroups

	Percentage answering 'yes' to:	
	Q.26	Q.27
All adult migrants	58	55
Type of job		
GP	57	63
Hospital doctor	59	53
Country of first qualification:		
UK/Eire	51	49
White anglophone country	56	61
Indian sub-continent	59	56
Arab country	69	47
Elsewhere	54	60
Present specialty		
Geriatrics	72	47
Other medical specialties	64	46
General surgery	67	51
Other surgical specialties	59	63
Anaesthetics	53	54
Radiology/radiotherapy +	47	66
Gynaecology	67	47
Pathology specialties +	53	53
Psychiatric specialties	47	61
Accident and emergency +	39	48
Other specialties	51	30
Year of coming to the UK		
Up to 1959	49	n.a.
1960-72	66	n.a.
1973-76	55	n.a.
1977-78	44	n.a.
Overseas-qualified migrants according to language test score:		
0-14	52	51
15-18	59	47
19-23	60	61
24-25	56	61
26-27	61	56
28-29	61	55

+ Low base for percentage (unweighted between 26 and 32)

Q26 Is there anything about studying or working in Britain that has disappointed you?

Q28 Is there anything about studying or working in Britain that is better than you expected?

Table A15   Attitudes towards training and experience obtained in the UK:
adult migrants and various subgroups

	Percentage answering 'yes' to Q.22/24:	
	Training	Experience
All adult migrants	**59**	**58**
Type of job		
General practitioner	51	53
Hospital doctor	61	60
Country of first qualification		
UK/Eire	64	65
White anglophone country	40	45
Indian sub/continent	59	58
Arab country	77	66
Elsewhere	48	57
Present specialty		
Geriatrics	47	55
Other medical specialties	61	63
General surgery	59	57
Other surgical specialties	57	59
Anaesthetics	75	65
+ Radiology/radiotherapy	69	75
Gynaecology/obstetrics	59	59
+ Pathology specialties	44	71
Psychiatric specialties	75	67
+ Accident and emergency	48	39
Other specialties	72	60
Highest qualification		
Membership/fellowship	71	64
Membership/fellowship Part 1 only	63	65
British Diploma	68	67
Other qualification	59	57
No qualification	46	51
Overseas-qualified doctors according to language test score		
0-14	49	51
15-18	61	59
19-23	57	58
24-25	66	67
26-27	64	60
28-29	58	50

+ Low base for percentage (unweighted between 26 and 31)

Q22/24 Have you obtained training/medical experience in Britain that you would not have obtained in your country of origin?

Table A16 Salary expectations and experience, by type of post and country of first qualification: adult migrants

Column percentages

	Total	Job type: GP	Hospital doctor	UK/Eire	Country of first qualification: White anglophone country	Indian sub-continent	Arab country	Elsewhere
Expected rates of pay:								
Higher in Britain	44	43	44	31	3	57	26	22
Higher in country of origin	16	8	18	9	82	5	27	21
About the same	16	15	16	4	9	15	24	25
No definite expectation	24	34	21	56	6	23	23	32
Actual rates of pay of hospital doctors								
Higher in Britain	51	58	48	19	2	65	37	38
Higher in country of origin	19	11	21	20	82	7	37	21
About the same	17	9	20	17	6	18	19	21
Don't know	13	21	10	44	10	10	7	21
Actual earnings of GPs								
Higher in Britain	25	27	24	13	1	31	21	17
Higher in country of origin	33	33	33	39	75	24	41	42
About the same	11	14	11	4	3	14	8	7
Don't know	31	26	32	47	20	30	29	34
Base: Adult migrants								
Unweighted	*1,016*	*273*	*743*	*61*	*66*	*661*	*111*	*117*
Weighted	*1,160*	*291*	*869*	*69*	*94*	*741*	*119*	*137*

Q16 Before you came to Britain, did you think that rates of pay for equivalent medical jobs were higher in Britain, higher in country of origin, or about the same in the two countries?
Q17 Do you now find that rates of pay for *hospital* doctors in equivalent jobs are higher in Britain, higher in your country of origin or about the same in the two countries?
Q18 Do you now find that earnings of *general practitioners* are higher in Britain, higher in your country of origin or about the same in the two countries?

Table A17   **Intended length of stay on coming to the UK, by year of coming: adult migrants**

Column percentages

	Year of coming to the UK:						
	Up to 1959	1960-1964	1965-1969	1970-1972	1973-1974	1975-1976	1977-1978
Up to 3 years	29	46	32	28	21	42	57
4-5 years	34	39	43	41	62	47	36
6-9 years	12	10	12	18	13	7	2
10 or more years	7	1	3	6	—	*	—
Permanently	18	4	10	7	4	4	5
Base: Adult migrants							
Unweighted	*137*	*107*	*193*	*130*	*203*	*196*	*50*
Weighted	*146*	*123*	*224*	*154*	*227*	*220*	*66*

NB: Informants who did not intend to stay permanently but had no definite expectation of the number of years have been redistributed proportionately to those who did have a definite expectation.

Table A18   **Actual and intended length of stay in the UK by year of coming to the UK: adult migrants**

Column percentages

	Year of coming to the UK:						
	Up to 1959	1960-1964	1965-1969	1970-1972	1973-1974	1975-1976	1977-1978
Has stayed longer than intended	59	80	79	44	20	5	—
Has not stayed longer than intended	4	5	5	33	63	86	73
Original intention uncertain	19	9	6	16	13	4	23
Intended to stay permanently	19	7	10	7	4	4	5
Base: Adult migrants							
Unweighted	*137*	*107*	*193*	*130*	*203*	*196*	*50*
Weighted	*146*	*123*	*224*	*154*	*227*	*220*	*66*

Appendix A

Table A19 Present grade of adult migrants who expected to reach registrar grade before leaving the UK, by year of coming to the UK

Column percentages

Present grade	Up to 1969	1965-1969	1970-1972	1973-1974	1975-1978
	Year of coming to the UK:				
General practitioner	49	51	5	1	—
House officer/Senior house officer	5	9	49	68	79
Registrar	16	24	42	25	17
Senior registrar/Medical assistant/ Consultant	27	14	—	5	2
Not known	3	3	4	1	2
Base: Adult migrants *Weighted*	*154*	*79*	*55*	*114*	*173*

1 This group is contained in the group in the previous column.

Table A20 Present grade of adult migrants who expected to reach senior registrar, medical assistant or consultant grade before leaving, by year of coming to the UK

Column percentages

Present grade	Up to 1964	1965-1969	1970-1972	1973-1978
	Year of coming to the UK:			
General practitioner	62	40	10	—
House officer/Senior house officer	2	2	14	40
Registrar	—	19	50	53
Senior registrar/Medical assistant	13 ⎤ 34	14 ⎤ 38	21 ⎤ 24	4 ⎤ 5
Consultant	21 ⎦	24 ⎦	2 ⎦	1 ⎦
Not known	2	2	2	2
Base: Adult migrants *Weighted*	*61*	*63*	*42*	*137*

221

Table A21   Progress in terms of further study and examinations, by country of qualification

Column percentages

	UK/Eire	White anglo- phone country	Elsewhere
		First qualified in:	
Whether progress as fast as expected:			
Yes	73	71	43
No	20	27	55
Don't know	7	2	3
Cause of slow progress:			
Examinations and study			
Not enough time to study	4	1	17
Failed examinations	2	3	7
Criticisms of examination system	*	5	2
Job difficulties			
Not able to get a good training job	1	—	10
Not able to get a job/the job I wanted	1	1	5
Few opportunities to train in most popular or chosen specialty	1	1	2
Other difficulties			
Family difficulty or commitments	3	1	5
Changed specialty or type of career	4	6	4
Personal difficulties/nervous breakdown	2	2	4
Difficulties of adaptation to a new country	*	—	3
Have not tried or studied enough	1	1	3
Discrimination, have not had equal opportunity	*	—	2
Work long hours to maintain standard of living	*	—	2
Lack of money/poor pay	2	1	2
Frequent job changes lead to insecurity	*	—	2
Got married and therefore changed plans	2	—	1
National or wartime service	4	—	1
Accommodation difficulties	*	—	*
Opposition to married women doctors	*	—	*
Other difficulties	1	7	3
Base: All informants			
Unweighted	*1016*	*73*	*892*
Weighted	*3382*	*104*	*1004*

Table A22 Qualification expectations (within ten years of obtaining MB), by type of job and country of first qualification (Qs 66 and 67)

Column percentages

	Total	UK/ Eire	White anglo- phone country	Else- where
All GPs qualified in:				
Expected to get further qualifications:				
Yes	69	65	(13)	91
No	28	32	(6)	8
Uncertain	3	3	(—)	2
If yes, what qualifications:				
Membership/fellowship	34	30	(4)	60
MS/MD	5	4	(3)	9
MSc	—	—	(—)	—
Postgraduate Diploma	33	35	(1)	23
Base: All informants				
Unweighted	*730*	*477*	*13*	*240*
Weighted	*1,923*	*1,649*	*20*	*255*

	Total	UK/ Eire	White anglo- phone country	Else- where
All hospital doctors qualified in:				
Expected to get further qualifications:				
Yes	89	87	89	95
No	6	7	11	4
Uncertain	4	6	—	1
If yes, what qualifications:				
Membership/fellowship	63	60	51	71
MS/MD	12	13	6	11
MSc	1	1	—	*
Postgraduate Diploma	17	16	24	17
Base: All informants				
Unweighted	*1,251*	*539*	*60*	*652*
Weighted	*2,567*	*1,733*	*84*	*749*

223

Table A23 **Proportion of hospital doctors working in a teaching district[1],**
by country of qualification and grade

Per cent

Grade:	British-qualified	Overseas-qualified
House officer	41	n.a.
Senior house officer	47	15
Registrar	54	21
Senior registrar	88	74
Medical assistant or Consultant	36	17

1 Including London postgraduate hospitals (BGs)

NB The base for each figure in the table is different, for example the base for the first figure in the first column is British-qualified house officers.

Table A24 **Proportion of hospital doctors in selected specialties who are working in a**
teaching district[1], by country of qualification

Per cent

Specialty	British-qualified	Overseas-qualified
General medicine	29	21
General surgery	46	5
Anaesthetics	40	16
Gynaecology/Obstetrics	53	22
Psychiatric specialties	51	20

1 Including London postgraduate hospitals (BGs)

NB The base for each figure in the table is different, for example the base for the first figure in the first column is British-qualified hospital doctors in general medicine. Unweighted bases are in the range 37 to 87.

Table A25 **Proportion of hospital doctors working in a teaching district[1],**
by country of qualification and language test score

Per cent

Language test score	British-qualified	Overseas-qualified
0-18	n.a.	14
19-25	38	25
26-29	47	28

1 Including London postgraduate teaching hospitals

NB The base for each figure in the table is different, for example, the base for the first figure in the second column is British-qualified hospital doctors scoring 0-18 in the language test.

Table A26 Proportion of hospital doctors working in a teaching district[1],
by country of qualification and highest postgraduate qualification

Per cent

Highest qualification	British-qualified	Overseas-qualified
Membership or Fellowship	49	29
Membership or Fellowship Part 1	52	15
British postgraduate diploma	28	15
None of these	42	20

NB The base for each figure in the table is different, for example, the base for the first figure in the first column is British-qualified hospital doctors having the membership or fellowship.

1 Including London postgraduate hospitals (BGs)

Table A27 Present job type and grade by age:
British and overseas-qualified doctors compared.

Column percentages

	Age:									
	Up to 29 years		30-34 years		35-44 years		45-54 years		55 years and over	
	British	Over-seas	British	Over-seas	British	Over-seas	British	Over-seas	British	Over-seas
Job type										
General practitioner	10	*	51	7	54	38	66	51	58	40
Hospital doctor	90	100	49	93	46	62	32	49	42	60
Base: All doctors										
Unweighted	*242*	*133*	*146*	*300*	*207*	*363*	*233*	*109*	*188*	*60*
Weighted	*672*	*153*	*493*	*349*	*723*	*406*	*826*	*127*	*668*	*72*
Grade										
House officer	28	4	5	1	—	1	—	—	—	—
Senior house officer	50	72	10	49	*	29	*	11	—	—
Registrar	19	21	41	39	5	36	2	8	2	7
Senior registrar	1	1	23	5	18	12	2	10	*	5
Medical assistant	—	—	—	—	—	3	2	16	2	30
Consultant	1	1	20	2	71	16	87	48	90	54
Not stated	1	1	1	4	5	4	6	6	6	5
Base: Hospital doctors										
Unweighted	*225*	*132*	*79*	*277*	*92*	*218*	*76*	*54*	*67*	*31*
Weighted	*603*	*152*	*241*	*326*	*332*	*250*	*279*	*62*	*278*	*43*

Table A28 Highest qualification by age:
British and overseas-qualified hospital doctors compared

Column percentages

	Up to 29 years		30-34 years		35-44 years		45-54 years		55 years and over	
	British	Overseas	British	Overseas	British	Overseas	British	Overseas	British	Overseas
Membership/ Fellowship	14	9	74	19	81	43	68	40	61	21
Membership/ Fellowship Part 1	11	11	6	19	5	13	2	5	4	2
Diploma	1	3	3	6	2	10	17	16	16	35
MD/MS/MSc	—	—	—	—	2	—	5	—	—	—
Any foreign qualification[1]	*	13	—	13	—	9	—	10	—	21
None of these	73	65	18	42	11	25	7	29	19	21
Base: Hospital doctors										
Unweighted	*225*	*132*	*79*	*277*	*92*	*218*	*76*	*54*	*67*	*31*
Weighted	*603*	*152*	*241*	*326*	*332*	*250*	*279*	*62*	*278*	*43*

[1] Not including Education Commission Foreign Medical Graduates (ECFMG) — the examination for medical practice in the USA.

**Table A29 Job type and grade, by highest postgraduate qualification:
British and overseas-qualified doctors compared**

Column percentages

	Highest postgraduate qualification:							
	Membership/ Fellowship		Membership/ Fellowship Part 1		British postgraduate Diploma		None of these	
	British	Over- seas	British	Over- seas	British	Over- seas	British	Over- seas
Job type								
General practitioner	11	18	39	10	84	50	59	25
Hospital doctor	89	82	61	90	16	50	41	75
Base: All doctors								
Unweighted	*271*	*235*	*70*	*110*	*198*	*129*	*477*	*491*
Weighted	*1007*	*265*	*187*	*126*	*689*	*144*	*1499*	*570*
Grade								
House officer	—	—	—	2	—	—	29	2
Senior house officer	3	11	31	36	4	26	42	62
Registrar	15	39	47	47	13	31	7	22
Senior registrar	12	17	4	7	5	3	1	2
Medical assistant	—	2	—	2	—	15	2	3
Consultant	68	28	18	6	68	22	14	4
Not stated	2	4	—	—	10	3	5	4
Base: Hospital doctors								
Unweighted	*238*	*186*	*49*	*98*	*39*	*64*	*213*	*364*
Weighted	*896*	*218*	*114*	*114*	*112*	*72*	*610*	*429*

**Table A30 Grade of hospital doctors, by language test score:
British and overseas-qualified doctors compared**

Number   Column Percentages

	Language test score:					
	0-18		19-25		26-29	
	British	Overseas	British	Overseas	British	Overseas
House officer	(1)	2	20	*	9	2
Senior house officer	(—)	61	22	39	19	13
Registrar	(—)	29	20	37	14	26
Senior registrar	(—)	2	1	8	8	13
Medical assistant	(—)	1	1	4	1	7
Consultant	(—)	2	29	7	46	40
Not stated	(—)	3	8	5	2	1
Base: Hospital doctors						
Unweighted	*1*	*255*	*43*	*300*	*463*	*120*
Weighted	*1*	*287*	*87*	*353*	*1539*	*144*

Table A31   Highest qualification, by language test score:
British and overseas-qualified hospital doctors compared

Number   Column percentages

| | \multicolumn{6}{c}{Language test score:} | | | | | |
| | 0-18 | | 19-25 | | 26-29 | |
	British	Overseas	British	Overseas	British	Overseas
Membership/Fellowship	(—)	13	41	30	52	42
Membership/Fellowship Part 1	(—)	11	8	16	7	10
Diploma	(—)	5	3	10	6	13
MD/MS/MSc	(—)	—	—	—	1	—
Any foreign qualifications[1]	(—)	15	—	11	*	14
None of these	(1)	55	47	33	33	21
Base: Hospital doctors						
Unweighted	*1*	*255*	*43*	*300*	*463*	*120*
Weighted	*1*	*287*	*87*	*353*	*1539*	*144*

1 Not including ECFMG

Table A32   Total hours spent working or on call in one week:
hospital doctors by grade and country of qualification (Q135)

Grade	British-qualified	Overseas-qualified
House officer	98	98
Senior house officer	86	92
Registrar	86	93
Senior registrar	85	88
Medical assistant	49	62
Consultant	88	88
All grades	88	90

NB The figures shown are means. For each cell in the table there is a different base.

Table A33 **Hours spent actually working in one week: hospital doctors by grade and country of qualification (Q136)**

Grade	British-qualified	Overseas-qualified
House officer	74	72
Senior house officer	64	66
Registrar	62	62
Senior registrar	55	52
Medical assistant	45	48
Consultant	49	51
All grades	57	61

NB The figures shown are means. For each cell in the table there is a different base.

Table A34 **Hours spent actually working in one week: hospital doctors by specialty (Q136)**

Specialty	Unweighted base	Mean hours
Paediatrics	53	60
Geriatrics	78	58
General medicine	128	66
Other medical specialties	63	58
All medical specialties	**322**	**62**
Orthopaedics	86	64
General surgery	127	71
Other surgical specialties	72	53
All surgical specialties	**285**	**64**
Anaesthetics	136	55
Radiology/radiotherapy	53	44
Gynaecology/obstetrics	106	66
Pathology specialties	63	54
Psychiatric specialties	114	50
Accident and emergency	52	51
Other specialties	71	52
All specialties	**1251**	**58**

Table A35   Number of mornings and afternoons off for study in a four-week period: junior hospital doctors, by grade and country of qualification (Q142)

Grade	British-qualified	Overseas-qualified
House officer	1.1	n.a.
Senior house officer	2.8	2.4
Registrar	2.0	2.1
Senior registrar	3.3	2.1[1]
Medical assistant	n.a.	n.a.
All junior grades	2.3	2.2

1 Low base (unweighted 33)

NB The figures given in this table are means.

Table A36   Contact with postgraduate tutor, by country of qualification (Qs 145-146)

Per cent

	British-qualified	Overseas-qualified
Postgraduate tutor not known	28	27
Number of hours spent with tutor per week (if known by informant):		
None	53	38
One	6	12
Two	5 ⎤	8 ⎤
Three	2 ⎟ 9	3 ⎟ 18
More than three	2 ⎦	7 ⎦
Not stated	4	5
Base: Junior hospital doctors		
Unweighted	*326*	*623*
Weighted	*903*	*729*

230

**Table A37   Number of hours spent per week in organised study,
by country of qualification (Q 148)**

Column percentages

	British-qualified	Overseas-qualified
None	14	27
One	21	21
Two	22	18
Three	17	11
Four or five	19	11
Six or more	8	8
Not stated	1	4
Mean hours per week	2.5	2.1
Base: Junior hospital doctors		
Unweighted	*326*	*623*
Weighted	*903*	*729*

**Table A38   Country for which hospital doctors intend to leave the UK,
by country of qualification**

Column percentages

	British-qualified	Overseas-qualified
Country of origin	7	81
Australia	15	2
USA	13	3
Africa	10	1
Europe	9	1
Canada	4	1
Asia	2	2
Other country	4	2
Don't know	37	7
Base: Hospital doctors who intend to leave		
Unweighted	*115*	*411*
Weighted	*318*	*480*

NB where the informant intends to return to the home country, this is classified as 'country of origin' regardless of what country it is.

Table A39   **Reasons for leaving the UK in future: hospital doctors who intend to leave, by country of qualification (Q.128)**

Column percentages

	Overseas-qualified	British-qualified
Training and experience		
Came to train and return	36	2
To gain experience of medicine in other countries	2	40
Links with home country		
Want to be at home/do not belong here	25	3
To rejoin family/relatives	18	3
Want to serve own people/my experience is needed at home	15	1
Want children to grow up at home	3	—
More respected at home/not a first-class citizen here	2	—
Have property at home	1	—
To accompany spouse	1	1
Career advantages abroad		
Better job/promotion prospects at home/abroad	18	10
More pay at home/abroad	9	18
Career disadvantages of Britain		
Difficult to progress in Britain	9	4
Financial incentives are poor in Britain because of taxation/NHS pay structure	3	17
Because of the state of the NHS (lack of money/resources)	2	21
Only have temporary registration	1	—
Dislike socialist attitude to medicine/phasing out private beds/little reward for merit and enterprise	1	6
Other answers	1	9
Don't know	*	1
Base: Hospital doctors who intend to leave Britain:		
Unweighted	*411*	*115*
Weighted	*480*	*318*

Table A40 Grade hospital doctors expect to reach before leaving the UK, by country of qualification

Column percentages

	British-qualified	Overseas-qualified
House officer	1	—
Senior house officer	19	5
Registrar	32	62
Senior registrar	19	19
Medical assistant	*	2
Consultant	13	6
General practitioner	4	—
Other answer	2	—
Don't know	10	6
Base: Hospital doctors who intend to leave		
Unweighted	*115*	*411*
Weighted	*318*	*480*

Table A41 Reasons for preferring to be a hospital doctor: General practitioners, by country of qualification (Q. 115)

Column percentages

	British-qualified	Overseas-qualified
Training or interests		
Would like to pursue my specialist interest/ this was my first choice	11	31
Have specialist training, would like to use it	14	15
Have academic interests/like lecturing/ dialogue with students or colleagues/research	25	4
Type of work		
Hospital work is more varied and interesting	19	12
Prefer to deal with serious illness	13	4
Dislike 'social medicine'/dealing with trivial complaints/being burdened with people's personal problems	11	9
Dislike administration/paperwork/routine of general practice	5	7
Shorter or more regular hours	10	10
Would prefer a hospital job if I could get a senior post in my chosen specialty	—	16
More job satisfaction (no further details)	26	13
Other answers	11	11
Base: General practitioners who would prefer to be hospital doctors		
Unweighted	*39*	*74*
Weighted	*123*	*81*

Table A42   Reasons for preferring to remain a GP, by country of qualification
(Q.115)

Column percentages

	British-qualified	Overseas-qualified
Freedom and Independence		
Greater independence as GP/you are your own boss/use your own resources	42	31
Hospitals are rigid/bureaucratic/authoritarian/ hidebound with administration/impersonal	15	12
Type of work		
Like involvement with people/treating people, not illnesses	41	38
More varied work as GP/cover a broader field of medicine	23	16
Like continuity of involvement with patients	10	13
Working conditions		
High pressure in hospitals	3	2
Lack of security in hospital jobs/no certainty of a job at the end of training	2	5
Difficult for a woman to get on in hospitals/ hard to combine with family commitments	4	4
I am not clever enough to be a specialist	1	3
Other answers	12	12
Don't know	3	5
Base: GPs who would prefer to remain GPs		
Unweighted	*428*	*165*
Weighted	*1486*	*179*

234

Table A43   Number of doctors in practice, by country of qualification
and years in general practice of informant (Q.96)

	Years in general practice:				
	Up to 5	5-13	14-23	24-33	Over 33
British-qualified informant					
Mean number of doctors in practice	4.4	3.8	3.9	3.6	3.5
Per cent in single doctor practices	4	7	6	11	23
Base: British qualified GPs					
Unweighted	*65*	*88*	*157*	*101*	*34*
Weighted	*241*	*299*	*547*	*347*	*115*
Overseas-qualified informant					
Mean number of doctors in practice	2.9	2.5	2.5[1]		
Per cent in single doctor practices	21	24	29[1]		
Base: Overseas-qualified GPs					
Unweighted	*85*	*103*	*39[1]*		
Weighted	*86*	*113*	*46[1]*		

1 Over 13 years

NB This table shows the practice size of practices to which a sample of individuals belong
— see note to Table VII.3

Table A44   Mean number of visits made to patients in an average week:
GPs, by country of qualification and age (Q. 104)

Age	British-qualified		Overseas-qualified	
	Mean number of visits	Unweighted base	Mean number of visits	Unweighted base
Up to 34 years	32.0	84	23.3	24
35-44 years	35.4	115	29.5	145
45-54 years	37.5	157	30.1	55
55 years or more	42.1	121	22.1	29

Table A45 Mean number of weekends on call out of every four:
General practitioners, by country of qualification
and number of doctors in the practice (Qs. 106-107)

Number of doctors in practice	British-qualified		Overseas-qualified	
	Mean	Unweighted base	Mean	Unweighted base
One	1.92	57	2.52	58
Two	1.39	60	1.66	75
Three	1.12	110	1.47	47
Four	0.85	106	1.53	36
Five	0.97	67	1.00	32
Six to ten	0.89	74		32

Table A46 Mean number of weekday nights on call out of every twenty:
General practitioners, by country of qualification and number of
doctors in the practice (Qs. 108-109)

Number of doctors in practice	British-qualified		Overseas-qualified	
	Mean	Unweighted base	Mean	Unweighted base
One	9.7	57	12.6	58
Two	7.8	60	7.8	75
Three	6.3	110	6.4	47
Four	4.7	106	5.3	36
Five	4.7	67	4.9	32
Six to ten	4.1	74		

Table A47 Mean hours worked during one week:
General practitioners, by country of qualification

Number of doctors in practice	British-qualified		Overseas-qualified	
	Mean hours	Unweighted base	Mean hours	Unweighted base
One	71.8	57	71.7	58
Two	58.2	60	75.2	75
Three	62.8	110	58.9	47
Four	62.8	106	71.5	36
Five	55.9	67 ⌉	60.9 ⌉	32
Six to ten	60.4	74 ⌋		

Table A48   Mean hours worked during one week: General practitioners, by country of qualification and years spent in general practice (Q.102)

Years spent in general practice	British-qualified		Overseas-qualified	
	Mean hours	Unweighted base	Mean hours	Unweighted base
Up to 5	59.2	65	70.0	86
5-13	66.4	88	71.1	113
14-23	64.6	157		
24-33	59.4	101	55.8	46
Over 33	47.5	34		

Table A49   Use of deputising services: General practitioners, by size of practice (Qs 110-111)

Percentages

Total	Number of doctors in the practice:					
	One	Two	Three	Four	Five	Six or more
Never used	59	47	53	51	63	79	63
Regularly used for:							
Holiday period	23	31	27	28	19	14	16
Normal weekends	27	35	35	34	22	15	19
Normal weekdays	26	34	29	34	23	12	23
Sometimes used but not regularly at any of these periods	5	2	4	3	3	4	9
Ever used	41	51	47	49	36	22	37
Not stated	*	2	—	—	1	—	—
Base: All General practitioners							
Unweighted	*730*	*115*	*135*	*157*	*142*	*89*	*84*
Weighted	*1923*	*219*	*297*	*433*	*405*	*262*	*289*

Table A50   **Number of job applications made before finding present job: hospital doctors by various factors (Q. 187)**

	Percent who made 7 or more applications	Mean number of applications
All hospital doctors	17	7.0
Hospital doctors born abroad by year of coming to Britain:		
Up to 1959	21	5.2
1960-64	9	4.8
1965-69	34	11.3
1970-72	37	12.7
1973-74	40	17.0
1975-76	43	19.5
1977-78	40	16.7

	British-qualified		Overseas-qualified	
	Per cent who made 7 or more applications	Mean number of applications	Per cent who made 7 or more applications	Mean number of applications
Present grade				
House officer	16	4.6	n.a.	n.a.
Senior house officer	7	3.2	52	22.8
Registrar	*	1.9	31	12.3
Senior registrar	*	1.7	23	5.0
Medical assistant	n.a.	n.a.	10[1]	8.7[1]
Consultant	10	3.3	11	3.3
Language test score				
0-14	n.a.	n.a.	52	25.9
15-18	n.a.	n.a.	45	21.1
19-23	n.a.	n.a.	37	14.1
24-25	9	2.9	26	7.4
26-27	9	3.5	23	7.1
28-29	6	2.8	22	8.8
Qualification				
Membership or Fellowship	7	3.0	29	11.7
Membership or Fellowship	8	3.3	38	16.2

[1] Low base (unweighted between 20 and 30)

Appendix B
Technical Data

The sample for the survey of doctors

The population to be sampled

The objective was to obtain a representative sample of GPs and hospital doctors in the NHS in England. While both British and overseas doctors were to be included, it was an important objective to obtain a large enough sample of overseas doctors for intensive analysis of this group. To achieve this within a total sample size of about 2,000 it was essential that overseas doctors should be over-represented: the imbalance would be corrected by weighting at the analysis stage.

In the case of GPs, only principals were included in the population to be sampled. The excluded groups (assistants and trainees) accounted in October 1976 for 5½ per cent of all GPs. In the case of hospital doctors, those with honorary contracts were excluded: these are largely doctors working in teaching and research. In October 1976 they amounted to 1,808 in England, or 6 per cent of all hospital doctors. Because the survey population was confined to GP principals and hospital doctors, certain other NHS doctors were excluded from it, namely those in the community health service, the blood transfusion service and in mass radiography units.

At October 1976, the population from which the sample was to be drawn was as follows.

	Total	General practi- tioners	Hospital doctors
Born in UK or Eire	34,764	16,886	17,878[1]
Born elsewhere	13,996	3,963	10,033[1]
Total	48,760	20,849	27,911

1 These figures are (close) estimates, because the breakdown of doctors with honorary contracts by country of birth is not known. Doctors with honorary contracts are excluded from the figures given and from the population to be sampled.

Outline of the sample design

The principle of the sample design can be stated very simply. Fifty Health Districts were selected with equal probabilities from the 206 in England. The population to be sampled was considered as falling into four groups: hospital doctors and GPs, in each case divided into those born in the UK or Eire and those born elsewhere. For each of these four groups, a constant proportion of doctors was selected across the 50 selected Health Districts. The proportions (or sampling fractions) were varied across the four groups broadly so as to boost representation of overseas-born doctors by a factor of 4½ to 1 compared with British-born doctors. Posts rather than doctors were considered to have been selected, so that where a doctor had left the post in connection with which he was sampled, his replacement was interviewed instead. Corrective weighting at the analysis stage restored the population proportions as between the four basic groups of doctors.

In order to explain how this general plan was put into effect, it is necessary to describe each stage of the sampling process in turn.

Selection of the sampling points

A list of the 206 Health Districts in England was prepared, with stratification by conurbation versus non-conurbation, teaching versus non-teaching district, region (or particular conurbation for the districts in the conurbations), and number of hospital beds in the districts. These stratification factors were taken in the order given. Fifty districts were then selected from the stratified list by taking a constant interval from a random starting point. All districts had equal probabilities of being selected, regardless of their size. The London postgraduate hospitals, which do not come within any health district, were separately provided for. They were divided into two (similar) groups, one of which was selected. At later stages, the sampling fractions for doctors at these hospitals were separately calculated.

Lists of hospital doctors

Hospital doctors may be employed either by an Area Health Authority (AHA) or by a Regional Health Authority (RHA), but never by the Health District, which was the unit chosen for our sample. DHSS centrally were able to provide lists of doctors by employing authority, but not by the particular district in which the doctors worked. Information about particular districts could only be obtained by the employing authorities (AHAs and RHAs). The method adopted was to obtain lists from DHSS centrally, to select a sample from this list in advance, and then to obtain further information about the selected doctors from the relevant employing authorities.

Computer print-out was obtained from DHSS listing hospital doctors employed by all the regions in England and by the 44 AHAs within which the 50 selected districts fell (in three cases, two districts had been selected within the same AHA). These lists were based on returns for 1 October 1976, whereas fieldwork was to take place about one year later than that. They were arranged by employing authority, and within authority by country of birth (UK, Eire, elsewhere) and by grade of post.

Selection of hospital doctors

Separate samples of UK or Irish-born and of overseas-born doctors were selected from these lists by taking a fixed interval from a random starting point. The interval, or sampling fraction, was different for these two groups (by a factor of about 4½ to 1) but otherwise constant across all employing authorities. Since the lists were heavily stratified (by employing authority, country of birth and grade of post) this was a rather efficient procedure.

The lists were then sent to the relevant employing authorities, with the selected doctors marked off. For each selected doctor, the authorities were asked to annotate the list to show in which district and at what particular hospital the doctor had all or most of his sessions. Where the listed doctor had left the post, the authority was asked to enter the name of his replacement, or to indicate that the post was vacant.

Only doctors who turned out to be working in the selected districts (or their replacements) were considered finally to have been selected. At the first stage of selection (before sending the lists to the employing authorities) we had to estimate how many of the doctors selected then would turn out to be working in the selected districts, and thus be finally selected. In practice, too generous a margin for error was allowed, so that one in four of those originally selected and who turned out to work in the selected districts were later rejected before arriving at the sample issued to interviewers. Taking this into account, the overall sampling fractions used were 0.116 for British or Irish-born hospital doctors, and 0.620 for overseas-born hospital doctors.

Lists of General practitioners
For every AHA there is a corresponding Family Practitioner Committee (FPC) to which GPs in the area are responsible. From DHSS centrally we obtained computer print-out listing GPs in the 44 relevant FPCs (principals only) and shown separately by country of birth, as in the case of hospital doctors. These lists did not show surgery addresses or telephone numbers. From each of the relevant FPCs we obtained a medical list, that is a list of all GPs in the area, together with their surgery addresses and telephone numbers (but not, of course, showing country of birth). The DHSS lists were then collated with the medical lists provided by FPCs so that each doctor could be classified according to the district in which his surgery fell, by reference to a map showing health district boundaries. Where GPs had more than one surgery, they were classified according to the location of the surgery where there seemed to be most frequent surgeries held. In some cases the GP, although responsible to a given FPC, did not have a surgery within its area. In such cases, the GP was classified as falling within the district of the responsible FPC which was nearest to his surgery.

Selection of General practitioners
The number of GPs in the 50 selected districts was then counted, separately for the UK or Irish-born and for the overseas-born. Two sampling fractions could then be chosen so as to achieve target sample sizes, and the sample of GPs was then selected by taking a fixed interval from a random starting point across all GPs in the selected Health Districts. This was, of course, done separately for GPs born in Britain or Ireland and for those born elsewhere. The sampling fractions used were 0.144 for GPs born in Britain or Ireland and 0.600 for GPs born elsewhere.

Analysis of response

The analysis of response is shown in Table B1. The first row of figures are the numbers selected after applying the sampling fractions that have been specified.

The response rate was substantially higher among hospital doctors than among GPs, even though hospital doctors were more likely than GPs to be unavailable for interview (for example because they were always busy). The reason for the lower response rate among GPs is that there was a very much higher level of refusals (33 per cent of British-born GPs and 31 per cent of overseas-born GPs refused to be interviewed). This high refusal rate among GPs seemed to arise because many of them expected to be paid to participate in the survey or had little sympathy with research of this kind. GPs were also not impressed by the fact that the project was financed by DHSS.

Table B1 Analysis of response

	General practice				Hospital service			
	Original occupant of post was born in:							
	UK/Eire		Overseas		UK/Eire		Overseas	
All posts selected	630		595		464		1,404	
	No.	%	No.	%	No.	%	No.	%
Unable to trace	16	3	19	3	17	4	61	4
Ineligible	5	1	7	1	3	1	13	1
Dead/retired, no replacement	2	*	4	1	—	—	3	*
Left, no replacement	6	1	3	1	18	4	70	5
All eligible posts	601		562		426		1,257	
	No.	%	No.	%	No.	%	No.	%
Refusal	198	33	172	31	50	12	176	14
Not available	4	1	5	1	23	5	70	6
On holiday	6	1	12	2	10	2	48	4
Sick	19	3	9	2	3	1	13	1
Other not interviewed	8	1	5	1	12	3	22	2
Interviewed	366	61	359	64	327	77	928	74

Replacement

In the case of hospital doctors, where the employing authority on annotating the original list found that a doctor had left the post, they were asked to enter the name of the replacement doctor or to indicate that the post was vacant. In the case of GPs we did not generally find out before attempting an interview that the listed doctor had left the post. In both cases, however, where the interviewer found that the listed doctor had left the post, she was instructed to interview the doctor who had replaced him unless the post was now vacant. Replacement was therefore used in both cases, though in the case of hospital doctors there were two stages at which replacement might occur. This was, in fact, an essential feature of the sample design, since it was inevitable that the lists would be somewhat out of date and that a substantial number of doctors would have moved from the post which had been selected. Replacement doctors were, of course, selected regardless of the fact that they might belong to a different group from the original occupant of the post, in terms of country of birth.

The actual extent of replacement is shown in Table B2. One way of summarising the table is to say that of all hospital doctors interviewed, 34 per cent were different individuals from those originally listed on the DHSS lists, whereas the corresponding figure for GPs was 8 per cent. The reason for this contrast is that hospital doctors move between posts far more frequently than GPs.

Table B2   Extent of replacement of the original occupant of the post

| | General practice | | | | Hospital service | | | |
| | Original occupant of the post was born in: | | | | | | | |
	UK/Eire		Overseas		UK/Eire		Overseas	
All informants	*364		359		327		931	
	No.	%	No.	%	No.	%	No.	%
Original occupant interviewed	323	89	342	95	238	73	595	64
Original occupant replaced by:								
British-born doctor	39	11	5	1	66	20	124	13
Overseas-born doctor	2	1	12	3	23	7	212	23
Total replacements	41	11	17	5	89	27	336	36

Weighting

Since 1976 DHSS statistics had been the starting point for the sample, these were also used as the reference point for reweighting at the analysis stage to restore population proportions. There were four basic groups within the sample which had been given different probabilities of selection (GPs and hospital doctors, in each case divided into those born in the UK or Eire and those born elsewhere). A weight had therefore to be applied to each of these groups to restore population proportions as shown by DHSS statistics. In carrying out this weighting we were, of course, dealing with posts rather than with individuals. Posts had to be classified according to the group to which the original occupant belonged, and weighted accordingly, even though a new occupant (who had been interviewed) might belong to a different group. The reason for this is that the chances of selection of the new occupant would be the same as if he belonged to the group to which the original occupant belonged.

The weights, unweighted bases and weighted bases are shown in the table below.

Table B3   Weighting factors

	Unweighted number	Weight	Weighted number
Hospital posts originally occupied by:			
British-born doctors	327	5.0615	1,655
Overseas-born doctors	931	1.0000	931
Posts in general practice originally occupied by:			
British-born doctors	364	4.2374	1,542
Overseas-born doctors	359	1.0076	362

Reliability of the English language test

A split-half reliability test was carried out on the 29-item language test (after the deletion of the item 'acid head'). The scores on the two sub-scales, consisting of the odd and even items, were highly correlated (r = 0.775). Correcting this correlation coefficient by means of the Spearman-Brown prophecy formula, we calculate that the reliability of the whole test = 0.873. Roughly speaking, this shows that only 13 per cent of the variance in the test scores is 'random noise': this is a very satisfactory level of reliability for a test of this kind.

Classification of specialties

The classification of specialties was done from the description given by the informant on a career history form (a part of the questionnaire that was self-completed). From this information it was not possible to make all of the distinctions contained in the DHSS classification, although the scheme that we have used is largely based on the DHSS scheme. The following list will make the survey classification clear.

i

Table B4   Classification of specialties used in the survey

Medical specialties
Paediatrics
Geriatrics
General medicine
Other medical specialties, namely:
    Cardiology
    Diseases of the chest
    Dermatology
    Gastroenterology
    Rheumatology/rehabilitation/physical medicine/physiotherapy

Surgical specialties
Orthopaedics
General surgery
Other surgical specialties, namely:
    Ear, nose and throat
    Genito-urinary/urology
    Neurology/neurosurgery

Other specialties
Anaesthetics
Radiology/radiotherapy
Gynaecology and obstetrics
Pathology specialties, namely:
    Haematology
    Histopathology
    Medical microbiology
    Clinical biochemistry
Psychiatric specialties, namely:
    Mental illness
    Mental handicap
    Any kind of psychiatry or psychotherapy
Accident and emergency
Other specialties

Although there are some differences of classification between the survey and DHSS statistics, there is a fairly good match in the distribution of doctors by specialty from the two sources, as shown in Table B5.

Table B5 Distribution of hospital doctors by specialty: survey and DHSS statistics compared

	Survey	DHSS statistics 1977
Base: all hospital doctors (England)	%	%
Paediatrics	5	5
Geriatrics	5	4
General medicine	12	13
Other medical specialties	6	11
All medical specialties	27	32
Orthopaedics	6	5
General surgery	10	11
Other surgical specialties	6	6
All surgical specialties	23	22
Anaesthetics	11	11
Radiology/radiotherapy	6	5
Gynaecology/obstetrics	8	8
Pathology specialties	7	7
Psychiatric specialties	9	9
Accident and emergency/other specialties	9	4

NB The column for the survey excludes that 4 per cent of hospital doctors for whom the present specialty is not known.

Appendix C
The Questionnaire
and Language Test

The questionnaire and the language test have
been reproduced in this Appendix but the
sheets completed by the informants during
interview, giving details of career history, are
not included. (These are the coloured sheets
referred to in the questionnaire)

Overseas Doctors in the NHS

IBM No. 430
77/78/79

CAREERS' IN MEDICINE

JN. 81404

Questionnaire Number _____
2/3/4/5

Interviewer _____

Date of Interview _____

Time of Interview: From _____

            To   _____

Interviewers Code No. _____

AREA NUMBER

AREA CODE

           6.   7.   8.   9.   10.   11.

ADDRESS SHEET SERIAL NUMBER

                            12. 13.

SAMPLE GROUP
      14.   15. 16.

(i) Sex:		(17.)
	Male	12
	Female	11
(ii) Age: STATE AND CODE _____		(18.)
	Up to 24	1
	25 – 27	2
	28 – 29	3
	30 – 34	4
	35 – 44	5
	45 – 54	6
	55 – 59	7
	60 – 64	8
	65+	9
(iii) Marital Status:		(19.)
	Single	12
	Married	11
	Divorced/separated etc.	0

(iv) Household composition:

        (STATE) Number of children aged 0-4   (20.)

        (STATE) Number of children aged 5-15   (21.)

        (STATE) Number of adults aged 16+   (22.)

        (STATE) Total No. in household   (23.)

(v) ASK: Do you have a religion? (IF 'YES') What religion?		(24.)
	None	12
	Islam	11
	Sikh	0
	Hindu	1
	Church of England/Scotland	2
	Roman Catholic	3
	Presbyterian/Baptist/Methodist/ Congregational/United Reformed	4
	Other Christian	5
	Jewish	6
	Other (STATE) _____	

(vi) HINDUS ONLY		(25.)
SHOW CARD G		
What is or was your caste?	Brahmin	12
	Vaisya	11
	Kshatriya	0
	Harijan/Sudra	1
	Other (STATE) _____	
	None	2

		SKIP TO			SKIP TO

CARD 1 (26.)

①

(vii) Are there any languages that you speak fluently apart from English? What other languages do you speak fluently?
(CODE IN GRID BELOW)

(viii) What language or languages did you speak at home as a child?
(CODE IN GRID)

(ix) What language or languages do you now speak at home?
(CODE IN GRID)

	(vii)	(viii)	(ix)
	FLUENT	AS A CHILD	AT HOME
	(27.)	(29.)	(31.)
English		12	12
Afrikaans	11	11	1
Arabic	0	0	■
Bengali	1	1	
Cingolese	2	2	⋷
French	3	3	⋽
German	4	4	◢
Gujerati	5	5	⋾
Hindi	6	6	⋴
Italian	7	7	⋼
Polish	8	8	3
Punjabi	9	9	⋺
	(28.)	(30.)	(32.)
Spanish	12	12	12
Urdu	11	11	11
Other (STATE AND CODE)			
_____	K	K	⋖
_____	K	K	⋖
_____	K	K	⋖

(x) INTERVIEWER'S ASSESSMENT OF INFORMANT'S ACCENT IN ENGLISH   (33.)

Strong accent	12
Definite accent	11
Slight accent	0
Little or no accent	1

(xi) INTERVIEWER'S ASSESSMENT: HOW EASY IS IT TO UNDERSTAND WHAT THE INFORMANT SAYS?   (34.)

Very easy to understand	12
Quite easy	11
Rather difficult	0
Very difficult	1

(xii) INTERVIEWER'S ASSESSMENT: HOW EASILY DOES THE INFORMANT UNDERSTAND WHAT YOU SAY?   (35.)

Very easily	12
Quite easily	11
With some difficulty	0
With considerable difficulty	1

(xiii) INTERVIEWER'S ASSESSMENT: WHAT IS THE GENERAL STANDARD OF THE INFORMANT'S ENGLISH?   (36)

Perfect	12
Not perfect but:- Good	11
Rather poor	0
Very poor	1

NOW COMPLETE INTERVIEW BY ADMINISTERING COLLOQUIAL ENGLISH QUESTIONNAIRE

251

- 1 -

		SKIP TO
1.	In what country were you born? (CODE BELOW)	Q.2
2.	UNLESS 'India', 'Pakistan' OR 'Rhodesia', SKIP TO	Q.3

IF 'India', 'Pakistan' OR 'Rhodesia'

Can I just check that the place where you were born is in India/Pakistan/
Rhodesia as it is now? (AMEND CODING FOR Q.1 AS NECESSARY)   Q.3

3. What country did your family come from originally?

	Q.1	Q.3	
British Isles	(37.)	(40.)	
England	12	12	
Scotland	11	11	
Wales	0	0	
Northern Ireland	1	1	
Eire/Irish Republic	2	2	
Other (STATE AND CODE)	3	3	
Indian Sub-Continent			
India	5	5	
Pakistan	6	6	
Bangladesh	7	7	
Sri Lanka/Ceylon	8	8	
Black Africa	(38.)	(41.)	
Kenya	12	12	
Uganda	11	11	
Zambia	0	0	
Tanzania	1	1	
Malawi	2	2	
English speaking countries			
Australia	3	3	Q.4
New Zealand	4	4	
South Africa	5	5	
Rhodesia	6	6	
U.S.A.	7	7	
Canada	8	8	
Arab countries	(39.)	(42.)	
Iraq	12	12	
Iran	11	11	
Syria	0	0	
Egypt/United Arab Republic	1	1	
Europe			
France	2	2	
Greece	3	3	
Poland	4	4	
West Germany	5	5	
Other Country (STATE AND CODE)			
	K	K	
	K	K	

			SKIP TO
4.	IF INFORMANT BORN IN BRITISH ISLES, SKIP TO		Q.8

IF INFORMANT BORN OUTSIDE BRITISH ISLES	(43.)	
Not counting short visits of less than 6 months, in what month and year did you first come to Britain? STATE:	(44.)	
	(45.)	
MONTH _____ YEAR _____		Q.5

5. How old were you at that time?   (46.)

(WRITE IN EXACT AGE AND CODE AGE-RANGE)

EXACT AGE [|]   (47.)

(48.)

AGE RANGE :-	Up to 10 years	12
	11 - 15	11
	16 - 18	0
	19 - 24	1
	25 - 27	2
	28 - 30	3
	31 - 34	4
	35 - 39	5
	40 - 44	6
	45+	7
	Not stated	9

Q.6

SHOW CARD A

6. Could you look at this list and tell me at what stage of your education or career you came to Britain?   (49.)

Up to the end of primary school	12
After primary school, before completing secondary school	11
At the start of undergraduate medical education	0
During undergraduate medical education	1
Immediately after completing the M.B. or its equivalent	2
Up to 2 years after completing the M.B. or its equivalent	3
More than 2 years after completing the M.B. or its equivalent	4

Q.8

Q.7

7.	IF BORN IN 'British Isles', 'Australia', 'New Zealand', 'U.S.A.' OR 'Canada' (Q.1), SKIP TO	Q.8

IF BORN IN INDIAN SUB-CONTINENT, AFRICA OR SOUTH-AFRICA (Q.1) AND CAME TO BRITAIN AFTER COMPLETING SECONDARY SCHOOL EDUCATION (**Q.6**)

Did you receive your schooling mainly or entirely in English, or mainly or entirely in another language?   (50.)

Entirely in English	12
Mainly in English	11
Mainly in another language	0
Entirely in another language	1

Q.8

- 3 -

ASK ALL

8. CODE BELOW THE GROUP TO WHICH THE RESPONDENT BELONGS:-   (51.)

        A.   Born in British Isles (Q.1)   12

    Not born in British Isles, came to Britain:-   Q.61

        B.   Before completing secondary schooling (Q.6)   11

        C.   At the start of or during undergraduate medical education (Q.6)   0   Q.9

        D.   After completing the M.B. (Q.6)   1

ALL RESPONDENTS IN GROUPS C & D

9. Why did you first come to Britain? PROBE. Were there any other reasons?

_____

_____

_____

_____   (52.)

_____

_____   (53.)

_____   Q.10

_____   (54.)

_____

_____   (55.)

_____

_____

10. Did you come to Britain chiefly in order to further your medical training or career or chiefly for other reasons?   (56.)

    Chiefly for medical training/career   12

    Chiefly for other reasons   11   Q.11

    Not stated   9

- 4 -

11. From what source or sources did you obtain information about medical training or careers in Britain before you came? PROBE: Were there any other sources? (57.)

_____

_____ (58.) Q.12

_____

SHOW CARD B

12. I am going to read out a number of possible objectives that you may have had in coming to Britain. In each case could you tell me, from the card, how important that objective was to you when you made your decision to come here?

READ OUT IN TURN REPEATING QUESTION AS NECESSARY:

		Very important	Quite important	Not relevant/ Not important
To get a job with better training opportunities	(59.)	12	11	0
To obtain a specific kind of training not easily available in your country of origin	(60.)	12	11	0
To get medical experience not easily available in your country of origin	(61.)	12	11	0
To progress faster in your medical profession	(62.)	12	11	0
To broaden your horizons by travel	(63.)	12	11	0
For personal reasons	(64.)	12	11	0
To improve your standard of living	(65.)	12	11	0
To make a fresh start in a country you thought you would prefer	(66.)	12	11	0
To escape from political or religious difficulties in your country of origin	(67.)	12	11	0

Q.13

13. Were there any particular difficulties in pursuing a medical career or getting medical training in your country of origin? (68.)

Yes _____ 12 Q.14

No 11

Not stated 9 Q 15

IF 'Yes'

14. What difficulties? (69.)

_____

_____ (70.)

_____

_____ Q.15

_____ (71.)

_____

_____

- 5 -

15. What advantages did you expect to get from coming to Britain to train or pursue a career in medicine? PROBE; What other advantages?

(72.)

_____

_____

(73.)

_____

Q.16

_____

(74.)

| NEW CARD | CARD 2 | (26.) |

16. Before you came to Britain, did you think that rates of pay for equivalent medical jobs were higher in Britain, higher in your country of origin or about the same in the two countries?

(27.)

Higher in Britain	12
Higher in own country	11
About the same	0
I didn't know	9

Q.17

17. Do you know find that rates of pay for <u>hospital</u> doctors in equivalent jobs are higher in Britain, higher in your own country of origin or about the same in the two countries?

(28.)

Higher in Britain	12
Higher in own country	11
About the same	0
I don't know	9

Q.18

18. Do you now find that the earnings of <u>general practitioners</u> are higher in Britain, higher in your country of origin or about the same in the two countries?

(29.)

Higher in Britain	12
Higher in own country	11
About the same	0
I don't know	9

Q.19

19. Did you expect to progress up the career ladder more or less quickly in Britain than you would have done in your country of origin, or at about the same rate?

(30.)

More quickly in Britain	12
Less quickly in Britain	11
About the same rate	0
No definite expectation	9

Q.20

20. Has your progress in medicine in Britain been faster than you expected, slower than you expected, or about what you expected?

(31.)

Faster than expected	12
Slower than expected	11
As expected	0
Don't know	9

Q.21

- 6 -

21. Do you think that your progress has been faster than it would have been in your country of origin or slower, or about the same? (32.)

Faster in Britain	12
Slower in Britain	11
About the same	0
Don't know	9

Q.22

22. Have you obtained training in Britain that you could not have obtained in your country of origin? (33.)

Yes	12	Q.23
No	11	
Don't know	9	Q.24

IF 'Yes'

23. What kind of training? (34.)

_____

_____ (35.) Q.24

_____

24. Have you obtained any medical experience in Britain that you could not have obtained in your country of origin? (36.)

Yes	12	Q.25
No	11	
Don't know	9	Q.26

IF 'Yes'

25. What kind of experience? (37.)

_____

_____ (38.) Q.26

_____

26. Is there anything about studying or working in Britain that has disappointed you? (39.)

Yes	12	Q.27
No	11	
Not stated	9	Q.28

SKIP
TO

IF 'Yes'

27. What has disappointed you?   PROBE: What else has disappointed you?   (40.)

(41.)

(42.)   Q.28

(43.)

28. Is there anything about studying or working in Britain that is better than you expected?   (44.)

Yes _____ 12   Q.29
No   11
Not stated   9   Q.30

IF 'Yes'

29. What is better than you expected?   PROBE: What else?   (45.)

(46.)

(47.)   Q.30

(48.)

- 8 -

SKIP
TO

30. When you came to Britain did you think that opportunities for postgraduate medical training would be better here than in your country of origin, or worse, or about the same?

(49.)

Better in Britain	12	
Worse in Britain	11	
About the same	0	Q.31
I didn't know	9	

31. Have you been pleased or disappointed by the opportunities for postgraduate medical training actually available to you *here*?

(50.)

Pleased	12	Q.32
Disappointed	11	Q.33
Not stated/Not relevant	9	

IF 'pleased'/'disappointed'

32. What has pleased/disappointed you? PROBE: What else about your postgraduate medical training *here* has pleased/disappointed you?

(51.)

_____

_____

(52.)

_____

_____

(53.)

Q.33

_____

_____

(54.)

_____

_____

33. At the time when you first came, did you intend to stay in Britain permanently or did you intend to leave after a while?

(55.)

Stay permanently	12	Q.42
Leave after a while	11	Q.34
Didn't know	9	

(56.)

IF 'Leave after a while'/'Didn't know'

34. For how many years did you intend to stay in Britain?

(57.)

STATE _____

Q.35

35. For how many years have you now been here in Britain?

(58.)

STATE _____

(59.)

Q.36

259

- 9 -

36. BY COMPARISON OF QUESTIONS 34 AND 35, CODE BELOW WHETHER OR NOT INFORMANT
HAS STAYED IN BRITAIN LONGER THAN HE/SHE ORIGINALLY INTENDED   (60.)

Has stayed longer than intended   12   Q.37

Has stayed same time as intended,
or not as long as intended   11

Don't know at Q.34 or 35   0   Q.38

IF 'Has stayed longer than intended'

37. Why have you stayed in Britain for longer than you originally intended?
PROBE: Was there any other reason?   (61.)

_____

_____   (62.)

_____   (63.)   Q.38

_____

_____   (64.)

38. Did you (originally) hope to have any particular medical qualifications before
leaving?   (65.)

Yes   12   Q.39

No, none   11

Didn't know   9   Q.40

IF 'Yes'

39. What qualifications?   (66.)

_____

_____   (67.)   Q.40

		SKIP TO

40. What grade of job did you expect to reach before leaving Britain? **(68.)**

Hospital Doctor:

House doctor	12
Senior house officer	11
Registrar	0
Senior Registrar	1
Medical Assistant	2
Consultant	3
Other (STATE)	

_____

GP: **(69.)**

Trainee	12
Assistant	11
Principal	0
Other (STATE)	Q.41

_____

Other answer (STATE)

_____

Don't know	9

41. Where did you intend to go from Britain? **(70.)**

Back to country of origin	12	
U.S.A.	11	
Canada	0	
Europe	1	Q.42
Australasia	2	
Other (STATE) _____		
I didn't know	9	

42. IF RESPONDENT IN GROUP D (Q.8), SKIP TO | | Q.47 |

IF RESPONDENT IN GROUP C (Q.8)

Did you already have a place on a British undergraduate course before you came? **(71.)**

Yes	12	
No	11	Q.43
Not stated	9	

43. Did you receive a grant or other financial support to cover your undergraduate training in Britain? **(72.)**

Yes	12	Q.44
No	11	
Not stated	9	Q.45

261

- 11 -

IF 'Yes'

44. From what source or sources?

(73.)

(74.)

Q.45

NEW CARD	NEW CARD 3

(26.)

③

45. Did you expect undergraduate medical training in Britain to be better or worse than in your country of origin or about the same?

(27.)

Better in Britain	12
Worse in Britain	11
About the same	0
No courses in country of origin	1
I didn't know	9

Q.46

46. Did you think that the undergraduate medical training you received in Britain was, in fact, better or worse than training you would have got in your country of origin, or was it about the same?

(28.)

Better in Britain	12
Worse in Britain	11
About the same	0
No courses in country of origin	1
Don't know	9

Q.51

ASK ALL RESPONDENTS IN GROUP D, (Q.8)

47. Had you already obtained a medical job in Britain before you came?

(29.)

Yes	12	Q.49
No	11	Q.48
Not stated	9	Q.49

IF 'No'

(30.)

48. How long did it take you after arriving to get a medical post?

Q.49

(31.)

WRITE IN _____

49. Did you have a grant or other financial support for any part of your first two years in Britain?

(32.)

Yes	12	Q.50
No	11	
Not stated	9	Q.51

IF 'Yes'

(33.)

50. From what source or sources?

Q.51

(34.)

	SKIP TO

ASK ALL RESPONDENTS IN GROUPS
C & D, (Q.8)

51. When you first came to Britain
were you married or single? (35.

Married	12	Q.52
Single	11	
Not stated	9	Q.57

IF 'Married'

52. Did your wife/husband come to
Britain with you? (36

Yes	12	Q.55
No	11	
Not stated	9	Q.53

IF 'No/Not stated'

58. Did he/she come to join you
later? (37.)

Yes	12	Q.54
No	11	
Not stated	9	Q.55

(38.)

IF 'Yes'

54. How long was it after you came
before he/she joined you? (39.) Q.55

WRITE IN _____

IF 'Married' (Q.51)

55. Did you have any children at
the time when you first came
to Britain? (40.)

Yes	12	Q.56
No	11	
Not stated	9	Q.58

IF 'Yes'

56. Did all of them come to
Britain with you, or some
of them, or none of them? (41.)

All	12	
Some	11	
None	0	Q.58
Not stated	9	

UNLESS 'Married' (Q.51)

57. Are you married now? (42.)

Yes	12	
No	11	Q.58
Not stated	9	

ASK ALL RESPONDENTS IN GROUPS
C & D, (Q.8)

58. Do you now have any children
younger than 16? (43.)

Yes	12	Q.59
No	11	
Not stated	9	Q.60

IF 'Yes'

59. Are all of your children now
in Britain? (44.)

Yes	12	
No	11	Q.60
Not stated	9	

60. Does you wife's/husband's/
family come originally from
Britain, from your own
country of origin or from
elsewhere? (45.)

Britain	12	
Own country of origin	11	Q.61
Elsewhere (STATE AND CODE)		
_____	0	
Not stated	9	

263

- 13 -

<u>ASK ALL</u>

61. At the time when you passed your MD did you hope to become a specialist, or a GP, or did you plan some other career? (46.)

Specialist	12	Q.62
G.P.	11	Q.64
Other career	0	Q.65
Don't know	9	Q.66

<u>IF 'Specialist'</u>

62. What speciality did you hope to pursue? (47.)

Accident and emergency	12
Anaesthetics	11
Cardiology	0
Clinical biochemistry	1
Dermatology	2
Diseases of the chest	3
Ear, nose and throat	4
Gastroenterology	5
General medicine	6
General surgery/Surgery	7
Genito-urinary/urology	8
Geriatrics	9

(48.)   Q.63

Gynaecology and obstetrics	12
Haematology	11
Histopathology	0
Medical micro-biology	1
Neurology/Neurosurgery	2
Paediatrics	3
Psychiatry/psychotherapy/mental illness/mental handicap	4
Radiology/Radiotherapy	5
Rheumatology/rehabilitation/ physical medicine/ physiotherapy	6
Other (STATE)	

I didn't know	9

(49.)

63. How long from graduating did you think it would take you to become a consultant (or the equivalent grade in your country or origin)?   Q.66

(50.)

WRITE IN _____

<u>IF 'G.P.' (Q.61)</u>   (51.)

64. At the time when you passed the MB, how long did you expect it to take you to become a principal (or the equivalent in your country of origin)?   (52.)   Q.66

<u>IF 'Other Career' (Q.61)</u>

65. What other career did you have in mind? (53.)

Community medicine	12
Medical research	11
Public health	0
Medical administration	1
Other (STATE)	

Q.66

<u>ASK ALL</u>

66. Did you expect to obtain further medical qualifications during the first 10 years after passing the MB? (54.)

Yes	12	Q.67
No	11	
Don't know	9	Q.68

(55.)

<u>IF 'Yes'</u>

67. What qualifications did you expect to get?

(56.)

68. In terms of further study and examinations, have you progressed as fast as you originally expected to? (57.)

Yes	12	Q.70
No	11	Q.69
Don't know	9	Q.70

- 14 -

SKIP TO

IF 'No'

69. What has caused your progress to be slower than expected? PROBE: Is there anything else that has slowed you down?

(58.)

_____

_____

(59.)

_____

_____

_____

(60.)

_____

_____   Q.70

_____

(61.)

_____

_____

_____

ASK ALL

70. Did you receive your undergraduate medical training at a <u>single</u> college, hospital or university or at more than one?

(62.)

Single institution	12	Q.72
More than one	11	Q.71

IF 'More than one'

71. At how many?

(63.)

(WRITE IN) _____   Q.72

ASK ALL

72. I would now like to collect some detailed information about your medical training and job history. First of all could you fill in this sheet which covers your undergraduate training?

HAND RESPONDENT BLUE SHEET. HELP HIM/HER TO COMPLETE THE SHEET IF NECESSARY.

NB. IF RESPONDENT HAS HAD UNDERGRADUATE MEDICAL TRAINING AT MORE THAN ONE INSTITUTION, ASK HIM TO COMPLETE ONE BLUE SHEET FOR EACH SUCH INSTITUTION.

Q.73

SHOW CARD C

73. How would you describe the reputation of the college <u>where you took your MB</u> among the medical profession in _____ (NAME COUNTRY) at the time you studied there?

(64.)

Excellent	12
Good	11
Average	0
Below average	1
Poor	2
Don't know	9

Q.74

- 15 -

		SKIP TO

74. Next, could you fill in your career history on this form starting from the first post you took after passing the MB and working through to your current post.

HAND RESPONDENT GREEN SHEET. HELP HIM/HER TO COMPLETE THE SHEET IF NECESSARY.

Q.75

75. Have you ever <u>sat</u> any medical examinations apart from the MB or its equivalent? (65.)

Yes 12 Q.76
No 11 Q.77

76. Could you fill in the details of all the medical examinations you have ever <u>sat</u> on this sheet?

HAND RESPONDENT PINK SHEET. HELP HIM/HER COMPLETE THE SHEET IF NECESSARY.

NB. THE RESPONDENT SHOULD FILL IN DETAILS OF ALL EXAMINATIONS HE/SHE HAS SAT WHETHER OR NOT THEY WERE PASSED.

Q.77

77. What kind of registration to practice medicine in Britain did you <u>first</u> obtain? (66.)

Provisional 12
Temporary 11 Q.78
Full 0
(67.)

78. In what month and year did you first obtain registration? (68.)

Month _____ Q.79

Year _____ (69.)

79. Has your registration status changed since this? (70.)

Yes 12 Q.80
No 11 Q.85

80. What was the next kind of registration that you obtained? (71.)

Provisional 12
Temporary 11 Q.81
Full 0

81. In what month and year did you obtain it? (72.)

Month _____ (73.) Q.82

Year _____ (74.)

NEW CARD	CARD ④	(26.)
		4

82. Has your registration status changed yet again? (27.)

Yes 12 Q.83
No 11 Q.85

83. What was the third kind of registration that you obtained? (28.)

Provisional 12
Temporary 11 Q.84
Full 0

84. In what month and year did you obtain it? (29.)

Month _____ (30.) Q.85

Year _____ (31.)

85. So can I just check that you now have provisional/temporary/full registration? (32.)

Provisional 12
Temporary 11 Q.86
Full 0

86. UNLESS "Temporary Registered" AT EITHER Q.77,80 OR 83, SKIP TO Q.93

IF 'Temporary Registered' AT ANY OF Qs. 77,80,83

Did you ever sit the Temporary Registration Assessment Board (that is, the TRAB) examination? (33.)

Yes 12 Q.87
No 11 Q.93

		SKIP TO

87. How many times did you sit the TRAB examination? (34.)

Once	12	Q.90
Twice	11	
Three times	0	
Four or more times	1	Q.88

IF 'Twice or more'

88. On the last occasion when you failed TRAB were you told that you could take the exam again in two months or ir six months? (35.)

Two months	12	
Six months	11	Q.89
Don't know	A	

89. On this last occasion were you told that you had failed on medicine or on the English Language, or both? (36.)

Medicine	12	
English	11	
Both	0	Q.90
Don't know	A	

90. Have you passed TRAB? (37.)

Yes	12	Q.81
No	11	Q.93

(38.)

IF 'Yes'

91. In what month and year did you pass it? (WRITE IN) (39.)   Q.92

Month _____

(40.)

Year _____

(41.)

92. How long had you been in Britain when you passed TRAB (WRITE IN) (42.)   Q.93

Month _____

(43.)

Year _____

ASK ALL

93. REFER TO GREEN 'CAREER HISTORY' SHEET AND CODE RESPONDENTS <u>CURRENT</u> POST BELOW. (44.)

GP principal	12	Q.94
GP assistant or trainee	11	
Hospital consultant	0	Q.124
Other hospital doctor	1	

- 17 -

ASK ALL GP's

94. Do you feel that you have had any problems or difficulties in practising as
a GP in England?

(45.)

Yes	12	Q.95
No	11	
Don't know	0	Q.96

(46.)

95. What problems have you had? PROBE: What other problems or difficulties are
you aware of?

_____

_____ (47.)

_____

_____

_____ (48.)

_____

_____ Q.96

_____ (49.)

_____

_____

_____ (50.)

_____

96. Including yourself, how many doctors are there in the practice, including
any assistants and trainees?

(51.)

One	12	Q.100
More than one	11	Q.97

WRITE IN EXACT NUMBER (52.)

97. How many principals are there in this practice?

(53.)

One	12	
Two	11	
Three	0	Q.98
Four	1	
Five or more	2	

- 18 -

98. How would you describe your working relationship with the other doctor(s) in this practice?
Would you call them excellent, good, acceptable or poor?

(54.)

Excellent	12	
Good	11	
Acceptable	0	Q.99
Poor	1	
Don't know	9	

99a. Could you tell me the national origin and ethnic group of each principal in the practice (not including yourself)?   COMPLETE ONE LINE BELOW FOR EACH PRINCIPAL (EXCLUDING RESPONDENT)

	National origin/ethnic group							
	White					Coloured/Black		
	British	Non-British						
Principal		From English speaking country	From Non-English speaking country	Indian	Pakistani Bangladeshi	Other Asian	Other coloured/ black	
1	A	B	C	D	E	F	G	
2	A	B	C	D	E	F	G	
3	A	B	C	D	E	F	G	Q.99b
4	A	B	C	D	E	F	G	
5	A	B	C	D	E	F	G	
6	A	B	C	D	E	F	G	

99b. And could you tell me the national origin of each assistant and trainee in the practice (not including yourself)?   COMPLETE THIS APPROPRIATE LINE BELOW

	National origin/ethnic group							
	White					Coloured/Black		
	British	Non-British						
Assistant		From English speaking country	From Non-English speaking country	Indian	Pakistani Bangladeshi	Other Asian	Other coloured/ black	
1	A	B	C	D	E	F	G	
2	A	B	C	D	E	F	G	
Trainee								
1	A	B	C	D	E	F	G	Q.100
2	A	B	C	D	E	F	G	

OFFICE
USE
ONLY

(55.)
(56.)
(57.)
(58.)
(59.)
(60.)
(61.)
(62.)
(63.)

ASK ALL GP's

100. Thinking of your current practice how many patients are there altogether on the list?

(64.) Q.101

(WRITE IN) _____

(65.)
(66.)

101 Roughly what percentage of these patients are coloured people, for example people from the Indian sub-continent, West Indians and Africans?

(67.)

(WRITE IN) _____

(68.) Q.102

269

- 19 -

		SKIP TO

102. How many hours did you work in the last full week, from Monday to Sunday? (IF ON HOLIDAY OR SICK, TAKE AN EARLIER WEEK)

(69.)

(70.)

(71.)   Q.103

(WRITE IN) _____

103. Is this more than usual, less than usual, or about the same as usual?

(72.)

More   12
Less   11
About the same   0   Q.104
Don't know   9

(73.)

104. How many visits to patients do you make in an average week?

(74.)   Q.105

(WRITE IN) _____

| NEW CARD | CARD 5 | (26.) |

⑤

105. How many patients do you see in the surgery in an average week?

(27.)

(28.)   Q.106

(29.)

(WRITE IN) _____

106. Are you ever on call at weekends?

(30.)

Yes _____ 12   Q.107
No   11
Not stated   9   Q.108

IF 'Yes'

107. On how many weekends in the average month?

(31.)

Less than one   12
One   11
Two   0   Q.108
Three   1
Four   2
Don't know   9

108. Are you ever on call on weekday nights?

(32.)

Yes _____ 12   Q.109
No   11
Not stated   9   Q.110

(33.)

IF 'Yes'

109. On how many nights out of twenty in the average four-week period?

(34.)   Q.110

(WRITE IN) _____

110. Does your practice ever use an agency night service?

(35.)

Yes _____ 12   Q.111
No   11
Not stated   9   Q.112

IF 'Yes'

111. At which of the following times is this service regularly used? (READ OUT REPEATING QUESTION AS NECESSARY)

	Used	Not Used	
	(36.)		
Holiday periods	12	1	Q.112
Normal weekdays	11	2	
Normal weekdays	0	3	

112. Do you do any hospital work in addition to your work as a GP?

(37.)

Yes _____ 12   Q.113
No   11
Not stated   9   Q.114

IF 'Yes'

113. How many sessions a week?

(38.)

Q.114

(WRITE IN) _____

- 20 -   SKIP
                                                                       TO

114. Would you prefer to be a hospital doctor, rather than a GP?   (39.)

                                                    Yes   12
                                                    No   11   Q.115
                                                    Don't know   9   Q.116

                                                               (40.)

UNLESS 'Don't know'

115. Why is that? PROBE: What other reasons are there for your preference?

_____

                                                               (41.)

_____

_____

                                                               (42.)

_____

_____

                                                                     Q.116

_____
                                                               (43.)

_____

_____

_____

_____

116. | IF INFORMANT IS A GP PRINCIPAL (Q.93), SKIP TO   Q.118

ASK ALL GP ASSISTANTS/TRAINEES (Q.93)

Thinking about the training and experience you are getting in this practice,
as a whole, are you very satisfied, fairly satisfied, fairly dissatisfied
or very dissatisfied?   (44.)

                                     Very satisfied   12
                                     Fairly satisfied   11
                                     Fairly dissatisfied   0   Q 117
                                     Very dissatisfied   1
                                     Don't know   9   Q.118

- 21 -

UNLESS 'Don't know'

(45.)

117. What makes you satisfied/dissatisfied with the training and experience you
are getting? PROBE: What else?

_____

(46.)

_____

_____

(47.)

_____

Q.118

_____

(48.)

_____

_____

ASK ALL GP's (Q.93)

118. Do you expect to remain in Britain for the forseeable future, or to go to
work in another country?

(49.)

Remain in Britain	12	Q.122
Move to another country	11	Q 119
Don't know	9	Q.122

IF 'Move to another country'

119. To what country do you expect to move?

(50.)

Country of origin	12	
Not country of origin:		
USA	11	
Canada	0	
Australasia	1	Q.120
Europe	2	
Other country (STATE) _____		
Don't know	9	

- 22 -

	SKIP TO

120. Why do you intend to leave Britain? PROBE: Are there any other reasons why you will leave Britain? (51.)

_____

_____ (52.)

_____

_____

_____ (53.)

_____ Q.121

_____ (54.)

_____

_____

_____ (55.)

_____

_____

121. In how many years from now do you intend to leave? (WRITE IN) (56.)

| | | |
|---|---|---| (57.) Q.122

ASK ALL GP's (Q.93)

122. Do you expect to continue working as a GP for the forseeable future, or to change to a different kind of job? (58.)

Remain a GP ..... 12 — Q.155
Change job ..... 11 — Q.123
Don't know ..... 9 — Q.155

IF 'Change job'

123. To what kind of job do you expect to move? (59.)

Hospital specialist	12
Community health service	11
Research/academic	0
Armed forces	1	Q.155
Blood transfusion service	2
Mass radiography units	3
Other (STATE)	
_____	
Don't know	9

273

- 23 -

ASK ALL HOSPITAL DOCTORS (BOTH CONSULTANTS AND OTHERS) (Q.93)

124. Do you feel that you have had any problems or difficulties in pursuing a career in the hospital service in England?

(60.)

Yes	12	Q.125
No	11	
Don't know	0	Q.126

(61.)

125. What problems of difficulties have you had? PROBE: Are you aware of any other problems or difficulties?

_____

(62.)

_____

_____

(63.)

_____

Q.126

_____

(64.)

_____

_____

(65.)

_____

_____

126. Do you expect to remain in Britain for the forseable future or go to work in another country?

(66.)

Remain in Britain	12	Q.133
Move to another country	11	Q.127
Don't know	0	Q.133

IF 'Move to other country'

127. To what country do you expect to move?

(67.)

Country of origin	12	
Not country of origin:		
USA	11	
Canada	0	Q.128
Australia	1	
Europe	2	
Other country (STATE)		
_____		
Don't know	9	

- 24 -

		SKIP TO

128. Why do you intend to leave Britain? PROBE: What other reasons?   (68.)

_____

_____   (69.)

_____

_____

_____   (70.)   Q.129

_____

_____

_____   (71.)

_____

_____

_____   (72.)

_____

_____

129. In how many years from now do you intend to leave? (WRITE IN)   (73.)

_____   Q.130

_____   (74.)

130. What grade or job do you expect to have reached before you leave?   (75.)

House Officer	12
Senior House Officer	11
Registrar	0
Senior Registrar	1
Medical Assistant	2
Consultant	3
Other (STATE)	
_____	
Don't know	9

Q.131

NEW CARD 6   (26.)
⊙

131. Are there any further qualifications which you intend to get before you leave?   (27.)

Yes	12	Q.132
No	11	
Don't know	9	Q.133

275

- 25 -

IF 'Yes'

132. What qualifications?

(28.)

(29.)   Q.133

_____

_____

_____

ASK ALL HOSPITAL DOCTORS (Q.93)

133. Do you expect to continue working in this same specialty for the foreseeable
future or do you expect to make a change at some point?   (30.)

Remain in speciality ____ 12 ____ Q.135
Change _____ 11 ____ Q.134
Don't know   9   Q.135

IF 'Change'

134. To what kind of job do you expect to move?   (31.)

Different speciality	12
General practice	11
Community Health Service	0
Research/academic	1
Armed forces	2
Blood transfusion service	3
Mass radiography units	4
Other (STATE)	

Q.135

_____

Don't know   9

ASK ALL HOSPITAL DOCTORS   (32.)

135. How many hours did you spend in the last full week from Monday to Sunday either
working or on call? (IF ON HOLIDAY OR SICK TAKE AN EARLIER WEEK) (WRITE IN)   (33.)

Q.136

(34.)

136. How many hours did you spend actually working in the last full week? (WRITE IN)   (35.)

(36.)

Q.137

(37.)

137. Is this more than usual, less than usual or about the same?   (38.)

More	12
Less	11
About the same	0
Don't know	9

Q.138

- 26 -

		SKIP TO

138. IF INFORMANT IS A CONSULTANT (Q.93), SKIP TO — Q.152

(39)

ASK ALL 'Other Hospital Doctors' (Q.93)

For how many beds are you yourself mainly responsible on a day to day basis? (WRITE IN) — Q.139

(40)

139. which of the following types of case do you regularly deal with? (READ OUT IN TURN REPEATING QUESTION AS NECESSARY)

	Deal with regularly	Not
	(41.)	
Chronic cases	12	4
Acute cases	11	5
Children	0	6
Old people	1	7
Men	2	8
Women	3	9

Q.140

140. Do you write correspondence and patient's notes regularly, quite often, occasionally or never?

(42)

Regularly	12
Quite often	11
Occasionally	3
Never	1
Don't know	9

Q.141

SHOW CARD D

141. In terms of its range and balance, how useful is the experience that you are getting from this job?

(43.)

Very useful	12
Quite useful	11
Not very useful	3
Not useful at all	1
Don't know	3

Q.142

142. In an average four-week period, how many mornings or afternoons do you have off for private or formal study?

(44.)

None	12
Less than one	11
One	0
Two	1
Three	2
Four	3
Five	4
Six	5
Seven	6
Eight or more	7
Don't know	9

Q.143

143. Do you have access to adequate library facilities in this hospital?

(45.)

Yes	12	Q.145
No	11	
Not stated	9	Q.144

IF 'No/Not stated'

144. Do you have access to adequate library facilities elsewhere?

Yes	1	
No	2	Q.145
Not stated	9	

145. Do you know who the postgraduate tutor is?

(46.)

Yes	12	Q.146
No	11	
Not stated	9	Q.147

IF 'Yes'

146 How many hours does he spend with you in an average week, either individually or in a group? (WRITE IN)

(47.)

Q.147

147. Do you have access to laboratory facilities for your own research?

(48.)

Yes	12	
No	11	Q.148
Don't know	9	

k

- 27 -

SKIP
TO

148. How many hours do you spend in an average week in organised study such as lectures, seminars and study meetings? (WRITE IN)

(49.)

Q.149

149. In general, what is your opinion of the opportunities for study in this post? Are they excellent, quite good, rather poor, or very poor?

(50.)

Excellent	12
Quite good	11
Rather poor	0
Very poor	1
Don't know	9

Q.150

150. What country does your consultant come from originally?

(51.)

Britain/Ireland	12
India	11
Pakistan/Bangladesh	0
Australasia/S. Africa/USA/ Canada/Rhodesia	1
(Other) Africa	2
Continental Europe	3
Middle East	4
Elsewhere	5
Don't know	9

Q.151

151. How would you describe your working relationship with him? Would you call it excellent, good, acceptable or poor?

(52.)

Excellent	12
Good	11
Acceptable	0
Poor	1
Don't know	**2**

Q.152

ASK ALL HOSPITAL DOCTORS

152. When they are in the hospital but <u>not actually at work</u>, do doctors belonging to different ethnic groups tend to mix together freely or do they tend to remain in separate groups?

Mix together	**3**
Remain separate	**4**
Don't know	9

Q.153

153. Are there any difficulties or shortcomings in working relationships between coloured and white doctors in this hospital?

(53.)

Yes	12	Q.154
No	11	
Don't know	9	Q.155

- 28 -

	SKIP TO

IF 'Yes'

154. What difficulties? PROBE: What other difficulties are there?

(54.)

_____

_____

(55.)

_____

_____

(56.)

_____   Q.155

_____

(57.)

_____

_____

(58.)

_____

_____

ASK ALL

155. Do you ever have language difficulties in communicating with other doctors?   (59.)

Yes	12	Q.156
No	11	
Don't know	0	Q.158

IF 'Yes'

156. With what ethnic groups do you have most difficulty in communicating?

White English speaking	1	
Indian	2	
Pakistani/Bangladeshi	3	
Middle Eastern/Arab	4	Q.157
Other (STATE) _____		
Don't know	9	

157. Would you say these difficulties are severe, moderate or slight?   (60.)

Severe	12	
Moderate	11	
Slight	0	Q.158
Don't know	9	

		SKIP TO
ASK ALL		
158. Do you ever have language difficulties in communicating with patients?	(61.)	
Yes	12	Q.159
No	11	
Don't know	9	Q.161
IF 'Yes'		
159. Does this happen frequently, quite often or rarely?	(62.)	
Frequently	12	
Quite often	11	
Rarely	0	Q.160
Don't know	9	
160. With what ethnic groups do you most often have language difficulties?	(63.)	
White English-speaking	12	
Indian	11	
Pakistani/Bangladeshi	0	
West Indian	1	Q.161
European	2	
Other (STATE)		
_____		
Don't know	9	
ASK ALL		
161. In your experience, do English patients ever dislike being treated by a coloured doctor?	(64.)	
Yes	12	Q.162
No	11	
Don't know	9	Q.164
IF 'Yes'		
162. Would you say this is common, fairly common, rather uncommon, or rare?	(65.)	
Common	12	
Fairly common	11	
Rather uncommon	0	Q.163
Rare	1	
Don't know	9	

		SKIP TO
163. Is this a serious problem for coloured doctors here, a slight problem, or no real problem?	(66.)	
Serious problem	12	
Slight problem	11	
No real problem	0	Q.164
Don't know	9	
ASK ALL		
164. I would like you to compare the level of competence of Asian and white British doctors in the National Health Service. First would you say that <u>on average</u> the competence of Asian and white British doctors is similar or different?	(67.)	
Similar	12	Q.166
Different	11	Q.165
Don't know	0	Q.166
IF 'Different'		
165. Which of the two groups do you think has the higher level of competence on average?	(68.)	
Asians	12	
White British	11	Q.166
Don't know	0	
166. Do you think that the variation of competence is greater among Asian doctors or among white British doctors, or is the variation about the same?	(69.)	
Greater among Asians	12	Q.167
Greater among white British	11	Q.169
About the same	0	
Don't know	1	Q.171
IF 'Greater among Asians' (Q.166)		
167. Do you think the proportion who are outstandingly good doctors is higher among Asians than among whites?	(70.)	
Yes	12	
No	11	Q.168
Don't know	0	

- 30 -

168. Do you think the proportion who are below a minimum acceptable standard is higher among Asians than among whites?

(71.)

Yes	12	
No	11	Q.171
Don't know	0	

IF 'Greater among white British' (Q.166)

169. Do you think the proportion who are outstandingly good doctors is higher among whites than among Asians?

(72.)

Yes	12	
No	11	Q.170
Don't know	0	

170. Do you think the proportion who are below a minimum acceptable standard is higher among whites than among Asians?

(73.)

Yes	12	
No	11	Q.171
Don't know	0	

ASK ALL

171. Suppose that two doctors with comparable qualifications and experience, one of them coloured and overseas-qualified, the other white and British-qualified, apply for the same hospital job in England.

SHOW CARD E

In this situation, what do you think will be the chances of the two applicants? Please choose a statement from this card.

(74.)

The two applicants will be offered the job equally often	12	
The white British-qualified applicant will be rejected slightly more often	11	Q.174
The white British-qualified applicant will be rejected much more often	0	
The coloured overseas-qualified applicant will be rejected slightly more often	1	Q.172
The coloured overseas-qualified applicant will be rejected much more often	2	
Don't know	9	Q.174

- 31 -

IF 'Coloured-overseas-qualified applicant rejected slightly
or much more often' AT Q.171

172. What makes you think that the coloured overseas applicant
will tend to be rejected more often? PROBE: Have you any
other reason for thinking the overseas applicant will tend
to be rejected?

(75.)

_____

_____

_____

_____   Q.173

(76.)

_____

_____

_____

- 32 -

| NEW CARD | CARD ⑦ (26.) ⑦ | | SKIP TO |

SHOW CARD F

173. For which of the following reasons do selection boards tend to reject coloured overseas-qualified doctors in your opinion? **(27.)**

They rightly put a lower value on overseas qualifications	12	
They wrongly put a lower value on overseas qualifications	11	
They rightly believe that the overseas doctor is less likely to be competent to practise in Britain	0	Q.174
They wrongly believe that the overseas doctor is less likely to be competent to practise in Britain	1	
They discriminate against colored overseas-qualified doctors on racial or ethnic grounds	2	
Don't know	9	

ASK ALL

174. NOW CODE THE RACIAL CHARACTERISTICS OF THE INFORMANT. (N.B. THOSE OF MIXED EUROPEAN AND OTHER RACES SHOULD BE CODED IN ONE OF THE NONE-WHITE GROUPS.) **(28.)**

White	12	Q.179
Brown/coloured	11	
Black/negroid	0	Q.175
Other non-white	1	
None-white mixed	2	

IF 'White' NOT CODED AT Q.174

175. Do you believe that you have yourself been rejected when applying for a hospital post because of ethnic or racial discrimination? **(29.)**

Yes	12	Q.176
No	11	Q.179
Don't know	9	

IF 'Yes' AT Q.175

176. Could you think back to the occasion when the evidence was most clear cut. How long ago was it? **(30.)**

Within past 6 months	12	
Within past year	11	
Within past 2 years	0	Q.177
Within past 3 years	1	
Within past 5 years	2	
Longer than 5 years ago	3	
Don't know	9	

177. What was the grade of the hospital post that you had applied for? **(31.)**

House officer	12	
Senior House Officer	11	
Registrar	0	Q.178
Medical Assistant	1	
Consultant	2	
Other (STATE)		
Not stated	9	

- 33 -

		SKIP TO

178. What makes you think you were rejected because of ethnic or racial discrimination on this occasion? PROBE: Had you any other reason for thinking that discrimination was involved?

(32.)

_____

_____

_____

(33.)

_____

_____

_____

(34.)

_____

_____

Q.179

ASK ALL

179. Suppose that two doctors with comparable qualifications and experience, one of them coloured and overseas-qualified, the other white and British-qualified, apply for the same job in a general practice where the other doctors are coloured and overseas-qualified.

SHOW CARD E

In that situation, what do you think will be the chances of the two applicants? Please choose a statement from this card.

	(35.)	
The two applicants will be offered the job equally often	12	Q.181
The white British-qualified applicant will be rejected slightly more often	11	
The white British-qualified applicant will be rejected much more often	0	Q.180
The coloured overseas-qualified applicant will be rejected slightly more often	1	
The coloured overseas-qualified applicant will be rejected much more often	2	
Don't know	9	

UNLESS 'offered equally often' AT Q.179

180. Do you think that this is because of ethnic or racial discrimination or because of other factors?

	(36.)	
Discrimination	12	
Other factors	11	Q.181
Don't know	9	

- 34 -

ASK ALL

181. Now suppose that two doctors with comparable qualification and experience apply for a job in a practice where the other doctors are white and British qualified. In that situation, what do you think will be their chances? (37.)

SHOW CARD E

Please choose a phrase from this card

The two applicants will be offered the job equally often	12	Q.183
The white British qualified applicant will be rejected slightly more often	11	
The white British qualified applicant will be rejected much more often	0	
The coloured overseas qualified applicant will be rejected slightly more often	1	
The coloured overseas qualified applicant will be rejected much more often	2	Q.182
Don't know	9	

UNLESS 'offered equally often' AT Q.18

182. Do you think that this is because of ethnic or racial discrimination, or because of other factors? (38.)

Discrimination	12	
Other factors	11	Q.183
Don't know	9	

ASK ALL

183. Have you ever applied for a job in general practice in Britain? (39.)

Yes	12	Q.184
No	11	Q.187

IF 'Yes' AT Q.183

184. Do you believe that you have yourself been rejected when applying for a job in a general practice because of ethnic or racial discrimination? (40.)

Yes	12	Q.185
No	11	Q.187
Don't know	9	

IF 'Yes' AT Q.184

185. Could you think back to the occasion when the evidence was most clear cut. How long ago was it? (41.)

Within past 6 months	12	
Within past year	11	
Within past 2 years	0	Q.186
Within past 3 years	1	
Within past 5 years	2	
Longer than 5 years	3	
Don't know	9	

		SKIP TO
186. What makes you think that you were rejected because of ethnic or racial discrimination on this occasion? PROBE: Had you any other reason for thinking that discrimination was involved?	(42.)	
_____		
_____		
_____	(43.)	
_____		Q.187
_____		
_____	(44.)	
_____		
_____		

ASK ALL

187. At the time when you got your present job, how many job applications did you make altogether?	(45.)	
		Q.188
(WRITE IN) _____		
188. In how many of these cases were you offered an interview?	(46.)	✱
(WRITE IN) _____		
	(47.) ↓ (76.)	

NEW CARD	CARD 8

COLLOQUIAL ENGLISH QUESTIONNAIRE   (26.)

SECTION I

I am going to read out some colloquial expressions for certain diseases and conditions.
In each case could you look at the card and tell me which <u>one</u> of the medical terms
corresponds to the colloquial one?   READ OUT SHOWING CARDS (i)-(x) IN TURN   (27.)

(i)	Pink eye	conjunctivitis	12
		albinism	11
		short sight	0
		Hordeolum	1
		don't know	9

(28.)

(ii)	Scurf	dandruff	12
		herpes zoster	11
		gonorrhea	0
		acne	1
		don't know	9

(29.)

(iii)	Thrush	nephritis	12
		diabetes mellitus	11
		tinea circinata	0
		monilia	1
		don't know	9

(30.)

(iv)	The change	menopause	12
		ageing	11
		puberty	0
		recuperation	1
		don't know	9

(31.)

(v)	Acid head	migraine	12
		meningitis	11
		take of L.S.D.	0
		halitosis	1
		don't know	9

(32.)

(vi)	Cissy	colic	12
		homosexual	11
		flatulence	0
		leucorrhea	1
		don't know	9

			SKIP TO
			(33.)
(vii)	Warts	enuresis	**12**
		erythema pernio	11
		parotitis	0
		veruccae	1
		don't know	9
			(34.)
(viii)	Boil	hydrops	12
		herpes simplex	11
		furuncle	0
		oedema	1
		don't know	9
			(35.)
(ix)	Ringworm	intestinal worms	12
		varicella	11
		variola	0
		tinea circinata	1
		don't know	9
			(36.)
(x)	Adam's Apple	testicle	12
		thyroid cartilage of larynx	11
		prostate gland	0
		breast	1
		don't know	9

SECTION II

I am going to read out some everyday phrases. In each case could you look at the card and tell me which <u>one</u> of the phrases on the card means the same as the one that I have read out. READ OUT STATEMENTS SHOWING CARDS (xi)-(xx) IN TURN

			(37.)
(xi)	Keep your hair on	Don't over-exert yourself	12
		Keep calm	11
		Keep yourself warm	0
		Stop shaving	1
		Don't know	9
			(38.)
(xii)	He is crackers	He is energetic	12
		He has a terminal illness	11
		He is highly intelligent	0
		He is insane	1
		Don't know	9

			SKIP TO

(39.)

(xiii)　I am whacked

am exhausted　12
have been beaten　11
am feeling elated　0
have lost all my money　1
Don't know　9

(40.)

(xiv)　She said she had the curse

She was in pain　12
She had a congenital illness　11
She was menstruating　0
She had tooth-ache　1
Don't know　9

(41.)

(xv)　I am all bunged up

ve got a headache　12
have eaten too much　11
have nasal congestion　0
have a bad cough　1
Don't know　9

(42.)

(xvi)　The patient said her husband often flew off the handle

He often became angry　12
He was often unwell　11
He often behaved as though he were losing his sanity　0
He often made impulsive decisions　1
Don't know　9

(43.)

(xvii)　The patient said he was a bit tight

He was rather anxious　12
He was slightly drunk　11
He kept his thoughts to himself　0
He was costive　1
Don't know　9

(44.)

(xviii)　The mother said her daughter was full of beans

She was overweight　12
She was difficult to control　11
She was growing fast　0
She was healthy and energetic　1
Don't know　9

289

		SKIP TO

(xix)   The boy said his girlfriend was in the club   (45.)

She was friendly and sociable	12
She was pregnant	11
She was a member of the fashionable set	0
She had contracted venereal disease	1
Don't know	9

(xx)   The husband complained he could no longer get it up   (46.)

He couldn't lift heavy weights	12
He couldn't get up in the morning	11
He had lost his enthusiasm	0
He was impotent	1
Don't know	9

SECTION III

SHOW CARD (xxi)

Could you take a look at this sentence? The word 'criticising', which has been underlined, can be replaced by the phrase 'getting at' - so the sentence becomes: 'My husband's always getting at me'. The verb 'get' has been put in brackets after the first sentence to show that it is used to make the substitute phrase 'getting at me'.

SHOW CARD (xxii)

Here is another example. The original sentence is: 'Paul invented these stories, about his parents'. Using the verb 'MAKE' this can be changed to the sentence: 'Paul made up these stories about his parents', which means exactly the same thing.

Here is a sheet of further examples on the same pattern. HAND OVER TEST PAGE. In each case, could you give me a fresh sentence that means the same as the one on the sheet, and uses the verb given in brackets? RECORD FOR EACH SENTENCE WHETHER RESPONDENT'S ANSWER IS CORRECT OR INCORRECT. (NOTE THAT IN SOME CASES THERE IS MORE THAN ONE POSSIBLE ANSWER.)

290

KEY TO SECTION THREE

		CORRECT	INCOR-RECT
		(47.)	(48.)
A.	My car has <u>broken down</u>.	12	12
B.	The nurse managed to <u>bring him round</u>.		
	The nurse <u>brought him round</u>.	11	11
	The nurse managed to <u>bring him to</u>.		
	The nurse <u>brought him to</u>.		
C.	I have never <u>come up against</u> this problem before.		
	I have never <u>come upon</u> this problem before.	0	0
	I have never <u>come across</u> this problem before.		
D.	I was in bed for a month but <u>I am getting about</u> now		
	I was in bed for a month but I <u>can get about now</u>	1	1
	I was in bed for a month but I <u>get about</u> now		
	Or similar sentences using 'getting around'.		
E.	You're making excellent progress.		
	<u>Keep it up</u>!		
	<u>Keep at it</u>!	2	2
	<u>Keep on with it</u>!		
F.	The patient was <u>looking forward</u> to his wife's visit	3	3
G.	I'm sure he stole the watch, but he <u>makes out</u> that he found it somewhere.	4	4
H.	I'm afraid you'll have to <u>put up with</u> the pain	5	5
I.	I'm feeling <u>run down</u>, doctor.	6	6
J.	Mike Yarwood <u>takes off</u> famous people in television programmes.	7	7
		(49.) ↓ (76.)	

✳

291

General Index

Compiler's note:

Acronyms have generally been avoided and names of interviewees omitted. Special attention is drawn to the list of tables to be found in the preliminaries and at the start of Appendix A. The general term "Doctor" has been preferred (appropriately sectionalised) to obviate synonymous and near-synonymous titles. The entry "Study" outlines the book's construction and conclusions. The letter-by-letter system has been adopted.